MW01166977

for the Long-Term Care Nursing Assistant

by

Joan Fritsch Needham, RNC, MEd

and

Barbara R. Hegner, RN, MSN

Delmar Publishers Inc.®

NOTICE TO THE READER

For information, address Delmar Publishers Inc.
3 Columbia Circle, PO Box 15015
Albany, New York 12212-5015

Copyright © 1992 by Delmar Publishers Inc.

Printed in the United States
Published simultaneously in Canada
by Nelson Canada,
a division of the Thomson Corporation

10 9 8 7 6 5 4 3 2

Library of Congress Cataloging-in-Publication Data
Needham, Joan Fritsch
    Pocket reference for the long-term care nursing assistant / by Joan Fritsch Needham and Barbara R. Hegner.
        p.   cm.
    Includes index.
    ISBN 0-8273-4840-1 (text)
    1. Long-term care of the sick--Handbooks, manuals, etc.
2. Nurses' aides--Handbooks, manuals, etc. 3. Nursing--Handbooks, manuals, etc.   I. Hegner, Barbara R.   II. Title.
    [DNLM: 1. Long Term Care--methods--handbooks. 2. Nurses' Aides--handbooks. 3. Nursing Care--methods--handbooks. WY 39 N374p]
RT120.L64N44   1991
610.73--dc20
DNLM/DLC
for Library of Congress   91-34652
                                                                      CIP

TABLE OF CONTENTS

CONTENTS

PREFACE

The number of elderly people in this country is increasing rapidly. While many of the elderly remain healthy and independent, there are others who need long-term health care. Providing this care is a complex and challenging issue. It is essential that the interdisciplinary health care team work together with the resident and the family to resolve the resident's problems.

The nursing assistant is a vital member of this team. It is the nursing assistants who give most of the direct care to residents in the long-term care facility. They have unlimited opportunities to influence the physical and psychosocial well-being of the residents. For this reason, they must be knowledgeable and capable of giving the care required.

This pocket manual was written to help nursing assistants in long-term care facilities to perform their assignments. It should be kept in an accessible area to be used as a quick reference source. It can be used by students during clinical practice and should also be helpful to experienced nursing assistants. Many procedures are learned in a nursing assistant course. The need to perform some of these procedures in the clinical setting may not arise for several months. This manual can be used as a quick review before beginning the task.

Most nursing assistants are proficient in basic nursing skills by the time they finish their training. For this reason, the basic procedures are not included. This manual has nine sections: Residents' Rights, Safety, Emergencies, Infection Control, Communications, Psychosocial Support, Abbreviations, Observing and Reporting, and Procedures. The information in these sections follows the requirements of the

Omnibus Budget Reconciliation Act of 1987 (OBRA). The sections (except Abbreviations and Residents' Rights) are presented in a guidelines format, beginning with the general and proceeding to the specific.

The sections on Residents' Rights, Psychosocial Support, and Communications are especially important. Residents in long-term care facilities have special needs. These sections provide suggestions for meeting these needs.

When an emergency occurs, there is not time to look up directions. The section on Emergencies is intended as a periodic review of life-saving techniques.

The Procedures section is in alphabetical order. Guidelines with beginning and ending procedure actions are presented at the beginning of the **A** section. These are not repeated with each individual procedure. A special symbol is repeated at the beginning and end of each procedure to remind the reader to implement these actions. Restorative nursing techniques are included in Activities of Daily Living.

This pocket manual is designed for quick and easy use. There is a beginning table of contents with the major headings of each section. A more detailed individual table of contents is presented at the beginning of each section. Section headings and content are listed in alphabetical order in the index. Thumb tabs on the side of the pages provide rapid access to needed information.

Nursing assistants are valued members of the interdisciplinary health care team. The more knowledge they have, the more they will enjoy their work with the residents. This results in a quality of care that all residents in long-term care facilities deserve.

ABOUT THE AUTHOR

Ms. Needham is a registered nurse certified in gerontological nursing. She has been involved in curriculum development, and classroom and clinical instruction for nursing assistants for more than 20 years at both the basic and advanced levels. More than ten years have been devoted to long-term care instruction.

Ms. Needham is the Director of Education at the DeKalb County Nursing Home in DeKalb, Illinois. She is also a continuing education instructor at Waubonsee Community College and Kishwaukee College, both in Illinois.

Ms. Hegner is a registered nurse with a master's degree in nursing and life sciences. She has taught nursing at basic and advanced levels for more than 35 years, established a curriculum for nursing assistants, and coauthored the textbook *Nursing Assistant: A Nursing Process Approach.*

Ms. Hegner is a professor at Long Beach City College in Long Beach, California, where she teaches students of nursing and life sciences, including adults planning careers as nursing assistants.

As a nursing assistant, you can assist residents to exercise their rights by being courteous and considerate, and by giving the resident choices. This is not a complete list of all rights. Included are those that nursing assistants can influence. Suggestions for assuring these rights are given. Familiarize yourself with the complete listing of residents' rights posted in the facility.

(NOTE: See Section F, Psychosocial Support, for additional information.)

RESIDENTS HAVE THE RIGHT TO FREEDOM FROM ABUSE

(NOTE: Immediately report to your supervisor any observed incidents of abuse by another resident, staff person, visitor, volunteer, family member, or other individual.)

1. Verbal abuse is:
   - Talking to residents in a sarcastic or rude manner.
   - Using slang or swearing.
   - Using gestures considered demeaning or obscene.
2. Sexual abuse is:
   - Using physical means or verbal threats to force residents to perform any sexual act.

A-1

■ Tormenting or teasing residents with sexual gestures or words.

3. Physical abuse is:
   ■ Hitting, slapping, pinching, or kicking.
   ■ Any physical contact that intentionally causes pain or discomfort.

4. Mental abuse is:
   ■ Making verbal threats to hurt or punish residents.
   ■ Humiliating residents.

5. Involuntary seclusion is:
   ■ Separating residents from other residents against the residents' will. (This may be permitted if it is part of a therapeutic plan and is documented.)

6. Physical and psychosocial neglect are:
   ■ Not attending to residents' physical needs for food, fluids, rest, activity, oxygen, cleanliness, shelter, and elimination.
   ■ Actions by staff that cause residents to withdraw, become agitated or depressed.

RESIDENTS HAVE THE RIGHT TO BE FREE FROM PHYSICAL RESTRAINTS

1. A physical restraint is any device or equipment that:
   ■ Residents cannot easily remove.
   ■ Restricts residents' movement.
   ■ Does not allow normal access to one's body.
   ■ Includes wrist/arm and ankle/leg restraints, vests, jackets, hard mitts, geriat-

ric and cardiac chairs, wheelchair safety belts and bars. Siderails may be considered restraints.

2. To avoid the need for physical restraints:
   - Care for residents' personal needs promptly.
   - Identify residents who are at risk for falling and monitor these residents. Alert other staff to help.
   - Check with nurse or physical therapist to see if residents can be instructed on safe mobility skills.
   - Report observations to nurse that may increase residents' risk of falling.
   - Report to nurse complaints of dizziness and problems with balance and coordination.
   - Maintain a calm, quiet, consistent environment.
   - Provide comfortable chairs for residents.
   - Cooperate with other staff to provide appropriate activities for residents.
   - Make sure residents have access to signal cords at all times.
   - Use siderails only if necessary.

(**NOTE:** See Section B, Safety, for caring for residents with restraints.)

RESIDENTS HAVE THE RIGHT TO PRIVACY

1. Close the door and pull privacy curtains when working with residents.
2. Always knock before entering residents' rooms whether door is closed or open.

3. Keep residents covered as much as possible when performing procedures.
4. Do not read residents' mail unless they ask you to do so.
5. Allow residents privacy for telephone calls and visitors.
6. Treat residents' rooms as you would their private homes.
   - Do not rearrange furniture without residents' approval, unless there is a medical or safety reason.
   - Do not go through dresser drawers, closets, lockers, or purses without residents' permission.
   - Be careful what you throw out when tidying the room.
   - Do not alter lighting, temperature, or ventilation in room against residents' will except for health or safety reasons.

RESIDENTS HAVE THE RIGHT TO CONFIDENTIALITY OF PERSONAL AND CLINICAL RECORDS

1. Any information about a resident is used only in caring for the resident.
2. Avoid talking about residents and/or family during lunch, breaks, or when off duty.
3. Read residents' medical records only when you need to in order to care for them.
4. If a resident or family member wishes to see the medical records, relay this information to the nurse.

RESIDENTS HAVE THE RIGHT TO MAKE CHOICES ABOUT ASPECTS OF LIFE THAT ARE SIGNIFICANT TO THEM

1. You are not directly responsible for this particular right. Learn which health care team members you need to contact to give residents these choices that can be related to:
   - Nutrition and eating.
   - Times of arising and going to bed.
   - Dressing and grooming.
   - Baths and showers.
   - Use of free time.
   - Visitors.

RESIDENTS HAVE THE RIGHT TO VOICE GRIEVANCES

1. Relay residents' concerns to the nurse in charge or other appropriate health care provider.
2. Perform all instructions you may be given for resolving the problem.
3. Never withhold care or attention from a resident because of grievances or complaints voiced by the resident.

RESIDENTS AND FAMILY MEMBERS HAVE THE RIGHT TO ORGANIZE RESIDENT AND FAMILY COUNCILS

1. Cooperate in assisting residents to attend council meetings.

2. Cooperate in performing recommendations of the council that are implemented by administration.

RESIDENTS HAVE THE RIGHT TO TAKE PART IN SOCIAL, RELIGIOUS, AND COMMUNITY ACTIVITIES

1. Relay residents' requests to appropriate health care provider.
2. Assist residents in preparations for attending any activities.
3. Arrange schedule so residents can participate in activities without interruption of care and treatment.
4. Respect religious articles and residents' worship practices.
5. Assist residents to make arrangements for voting in all elections.

MARRIED COUPLES HAVE THE RIGHT TO SHARE A ROOM

1. Respect privacy at all times.
2. Arrange for times without interruptions.
3. Understand the couple's need for intimacy and closeness.

RESIDENTS HAVE THE RIGHT TO USE PERSONAL POSSESSIONS AND FURNISHINGS UNLESS THIS INTERFERES WITH HEALTH OR SAFETY

1. Encourage residents to display pictures and family photos.
2. Assist resident to arrange personal items.
3. Request maintenance department to hang pictures or put up shelves for displaying mementos.
4. Treat residents' possessions with respect.
5. Display interest in family photos and mementos.

In summary, the resident has the right to an environment that:

■ promotes maintenance or enhancement of quality of life
■ promotes dignity and respect in full recognition of each resident's individuality
■ is safe, clean, comfortable and homelike, and
■ helps the resident maintain the highest practicable physical, mental, and psychological well-being.

SECTION B

Safety

B

TABLE OF CONTENTS

SECTION B: SAFETY

1. GENERAL GUIDELINES FOR SAFETY

Body Mechanics

Prevent fatigue and body injury by using proper body mechanics at all times:

1. Maintain good standing posture:
    - Feet flat on floor, separated about 12 inches and knees slightly bent.
    - Arms at sides.
    - Back straight.
    - Abdominal muscles tightened.
2. Basic rules for lifting:
    - Keep your back straight.
    - Keep your feet separated to provide good base of support.
    - Bend from hips and knees. Do not bend from waist, Figure B-1.
    - Get close to object or resident.
    - Use the weight of your body to help push or pull object.
    - Use the strongest muscles to do the job.
      — Flexor muscles are stronger than extensor muscles so it is easier to bring the resident toward you than to lift the resident away from you.
      — Leg muscles are stronger than back muscles.
    - Avoid twisting your body as you work.
    - Avoid bending for long periods of time.
    - Hold heavy objects close to your body.

(**NOTE:** An incident report should be completed
promptly after any incident involving residents, staff, or visitors.)

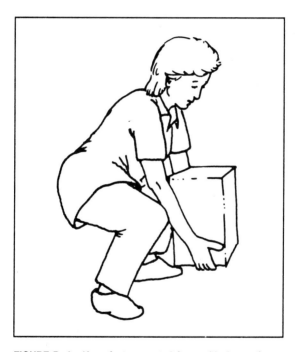

FIGURE B-1. Keep feet separated for a wide base of support, bend knees, and keep back straight. *(From Caldwell
and Hegner,* Nursing Assistant, A Nursing Process Approach,
5th Edition, 1989, Delmar Publishers Inc.)

Equipment

1. Beds
   - ■ Raise to comfortable working height when giving resident care.
   - ■ Put in lowest horizontal position when you are finished giving care.
   - ■ Make sure gatch handles on manually operated beds do not stick out.
   - ■ Raise siderails if ordered, and check for security.
   - ■ Do not attach restraints, drainage bags, or tubing to siderails.

2. Signal cords (call lights)
   - ■ Check call lights to make sure they are in working order.
   - ■ Residents must always have access to staff. If they are physically or mentally unable to use signal cord, an alternative method must be used, and residents must have frequent monitoring.
   - ■ Answer call lights promptly.

3. Other Equipment
   - ■ Use equipment only if you know how to correctly use it.
   - ■ Report needed repairs promptly.
     - — Lost screws
     - — Frayed straps or cords
     - — Loose wheels
     - — Broken control knobs
     - — Latches that do not hook
     - — Siderails that do not fasten correctly

— Missing feet on canes, crutches, or walkers.
- Dispose of needles and blades in proper containers.
- Never handle broken bits of glass with your hands. Use forceps or several sheets of moist paper towels.

Other Safety Measures

1. Keep all chemicals in locked cupboards.
2. Use only nonpoisonous plants in facility.
3. Keep all scissors, razors, and knives in safe places.
4. Check water temperature before using for baths or treatments.
5. Check temperature of food on residents' trays.
6. Observe residents while they are eating for signs of choking and aspiration.
7. Take special safety precautions for residents with dementia.
8. Be sure that you are aware of evacuation procedures:
   - Read disaster plan.
   - Participate in disaster drills.
   - Know the whereabouts of residents in your care.
   - Know the method of transport for residents in your care.
   - Know emergency exit routes.

2. GUIDELINES FOR RESIDENT SAFETY

Preventing Falls

1. Avoid obstructing open areas with supplies and equipment.
2. Immediately wipe up spills.
3. Encourage residents to use rails along corridor walls when walking.
4. Observe ambulatory residents for signs of weakness, fatigue, dizziness, and loss of balance.
5. Provide adequate lighting in all resident areas.
6. Eliminate noise and other environmental distractions.
7. Do not leave residents alone in tub or shower.
8. Care for residents' personal needs promptly.

Use of Restraints

1. Use restraints only when all alternatives are unsuccessful.
2. Try least restrictive device first.
3. Apply restraints according to manufacturer's directions.
4. Make sure restraint is in good condition and is the right size.
5. Tie restraint straps with slip knots for quick release in emergency.
6. Check residents in restraints at least every 30 minutes.
7. Release restraints every two hours:
    ■ Assist resident to stand and ambulate if possible.

- ■ If resident cannot do this, give passive range of motion exercises.
- ■ Take resident to bathroom.
- ■ If resident is incontinent, change clothing, chair pads or bedding and give skin care.
- ■ Check resident for signs of skin breakdown or irritation.
- ■ Change resident's position.
8. Give resident fluids regularly.
9. Place call light within resident's easy reach.

Moving and Transferring Residents

1. Never use a footstool to help a resident get in or out of bed.
2. Lock wheels of all transfer vehicles; beds, stretchers, and wheelchairs.
3. Check care plan for correct transfer method. If resident's condition has weakened, you may need to use another method. Check with nurse for instructions.
4. Use transfer (gait) belt correctly.
5. Two people should be present for a transfer with a mechanical lift.
6. Check resident's clothing for slacks that are too long and for untied shoelaces.
7. Assist resident to put on sturdy well-fitting shoes with nonslip soles before transferring or ambulating.
8. Allow resident to sit on edge of bed before getting up, to prevent dizziness.
9. Do not allow resident to place his/her hands/arms on your body while you are moving him/her.

10. Use turning sheets for moving residents in bed.
11. Check condition of canes, walkers, and wheelchairs regularly.
12. Be sure residents use canes, walkers, and wheelchairs properly and safely.

Transporting Resident by Stretcher

1. If resident has IVs or drainage tubes:
   - Keep IV bag/bottle above infusion site.
   - Keep drainage bags/bottles below drainage sites.
   - Keep tubes free of kinking or twisting.
   - Keep tubes free of stress at all times.
2. Check to see if resident's chart is to accompany resident.
3. Assume position at resident's head and push stretcher.
   - Stay to right of corridors.
   - Back down slanted ramps and through doorways.
   - Be careful when approaching intersecting hallways.
   - Back into elevators.
4. Transport resident to assigned area. *Do not leave resident alone.* Wait until another health care provider assumes responsibility for resident's care.
5. Return to unit unless instructed to wait.

Transporting Resident by Wheelchair

1. Position wheelchair beside bed on resident's strongest side.

2. Lock wheelchair wheels and raise or remove foot pedals.
3. Follow procedure for transferring resident from bed to chair (see Section I, Procedures).
4. Once seated, cover resident with lap robe. Be sure it doesn't drag on floor.
5. Replace foot pedals. Secure with foot straps if chair has them.
6. Unlock wheels.
7. When resident is in wheelchair:
   - Check for lap robes or blankets that can catch in the wheels.
   - Check resident's feet to be sure they don't drag under wheelchair.
   - Check resident's arms so they don't hang over arms of wheelchair.
   - Remind resident to avoid leaning forward when sitting in wheelchair.
   - Remember to put up foot pedals when resident is getting out of wheelchair.
8. Guide wheelchair from behind, performing these precautions:
   - Stay to right of corridors.
   - Be careful when approaching intersecting hallways.
   - Back down slanted ramps.
   - Back in and out of elevators and doorways, turning your head to assure clearance.
   - Once in the elevator, turn wheelchair so resident's back is toward the door.
9. Check to see if chart is to accompany resident.
10. Transport resident to assigned area. *Do not leave resident alone.* Wait until another

health care provider assumes responsibility
for resident.
11. Unless instructed to wait, return to unit.

3. GUIDELINES FOR FIRE SAFETY

1. Know:
    ■ Facility fire procedures.
    ■ Evacuation routes.
    ■ Location of extinguishers, fire alarms,
      fire doors, and fire escapes.
2. Participate in facility fire drills.
3. Be alert to fire hazards and report:
    ■ Frayed electrical wires.
    ■ Overloaded circuits.
    ■ Improperly grounded plugs.
    ■ Accumulated clutter.
    ■ Improper protection during oxygen
      therapy.
    ■ Uncontrolled smoking.
    ■ Matches and cigarette lighters.
    ■ Unsafe smoking habits of staff, residents,
      or visitors.
    ■ Oily rags and paint rags.
4. Remember the **RACE** system if fire occurs:
    ■ **Remove** all residents, personnel, and
      other people in the immediate vicinity of
      the fire.
    ■ **Activate** the alarm and notify other staff
      members that a fire exists.
    ■ **Contain** the fire and smoke by closing all
      doors in the area.
    ■ **Extinguish** the fire, if it is very small, or
      allow fire department to extinguish fire.

TABLE OF CONTENTS

SECTION C: EMERGENCIES

1. GENERAL GUIDELINES FOR ALL EMERGENCIES

1. Remain calm.
2. Ask someone nearby to summon the nurse.
3. Do not leave a resident who needs urgent care to get help yourself.
4. Do not move resident if you do not have to.
5. Do not allow resident to get up and walk.
6. While help is on the way, observe resident for:
   - Degree of consciousness.
   - Airway/breathing capability.
   - Rate, strength, and regularity of heartbeat.
   - Signs of bleeding.
   - Signs of shock.
   - Other injuries.

2. GUIDELINES FOR CPR (Cardiopulmonary Resuscitation) AND AIRWAY OBSTRUCTION

1. Federal regulations require all residents to have directives on their medical records that indicate whether CPR should be administered. Be sure that you know at all times the status of these directives on the residents you care for.
2. Know procedure for handling a cardiac arrest at your facility.
3. Know location of emergency cart.
4. Know location and use of disposable face shields.
5. *Do not attempt to do CPR unless you have completed an approved course and are qualified to do CPR.*

CPR (One Person) (For Adult Victim)

1. Call for the nurse.
2. Position resident on back.
3. Kneel beside resident's shoulder and open airway with head-tilt/chin-lift method.
4. Look, listen, and feel for breathing, for 3-5 seconds (Figure C-1).

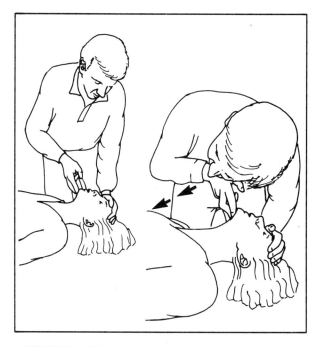

FIGURE C-1. Tilt head back. Listen for breath sounds and watch for chest movements. *(From Caldwell and Hegner,* Nursing Assistant, A Nursing Process Approach, *5th Edition, 1989, Delmar Publishers Inc.)*

5. Maintain airway with head-tilt/chin-lift method (Figure C-2).

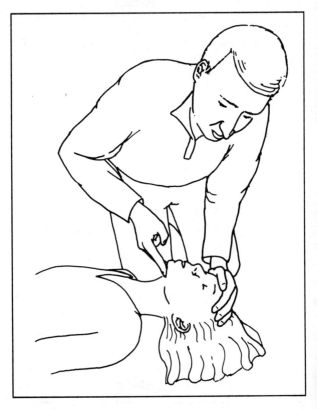

FIGURE C-2. Press down on forehead while lifting chin up with fingertips of other hand. *(From Caldwell and Hegner,* Nursing Assistant, A Nursing Process Approach, *5th Edition, 1989, Delmar Publishers Inc.)*

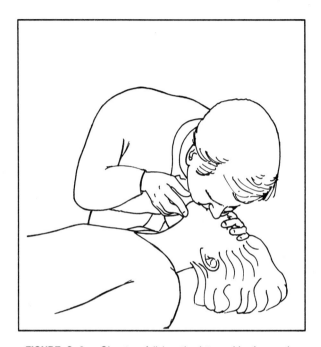

FIGURE C-3.   Give two full breaths into resident's mouth. *(From Caldwell and Hegner,* Nursing Assistant, A Nursing Process Approach, *5th Edition, 1989, Delmar Publishers Inc.)*

6. If there is no sign of breathing, begin ventilations:
   ■ Seal your mouth over resident's mouth.
   ■ Pinch nose closed.
   ■ Give two full breaths into resident's mouth (Figure C-3).

7. Observe chest rise and allow deflation between breaths (Figure C-4).
8. Check for carotid pulse on near side of resident for 5-10 seconds (Figure C-5).

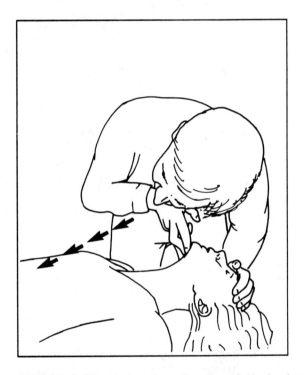

FIGURE C-4. Observe chest rise and fall. *(From Caldwell and Hegner, Nursing Assistant, A Nursing Process Approach, 5th Edition, 1989, Delmar Publishers Inc.)*

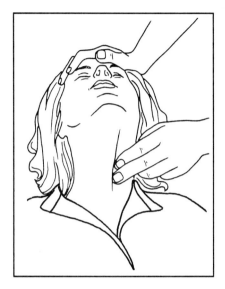

FIGURE C-5. Locate carotid pulse. *(From Caldwell and Hegner,* Nursing Assistant, A Nursing Process Approach, *5th Edition, 1989, Delmar Publishers Inc.)*

9. If pulse is present, continue with ventilations at rate of one every five seconds (12 times per minute).
10. If pulse is absent, begin compressions:
    ■ Find landmark by tracing along rib cage to sternal notch (Figure C-6).
    ■ Place middle finger in notch with index finger beside it (Figure C-7).

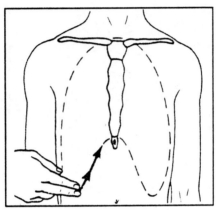

FIGURE C-6. Trace along rib cage to notch. *(From Caldwell and Hegner, Nursing Assistant, A Nursing Process Approach, 5th Edition, 1989, Delmar Publishers Inc.)*

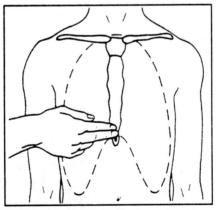

FIGURE C-7. Place middle finger on notch with index finger beside it. *(From Caldwell and Hegner, Nursing Assistant, A Nursing Process Approach, 5th Edition, 1989, Delmar Publishers Inc.)*

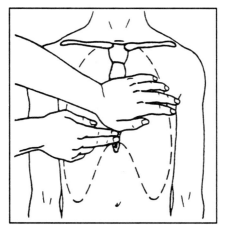

FIGURE C-8. Position other hand, placing it beside the index finger. *(From Caldwell and Hegner,* Nursing Assistant, A Nursing Process Approach, *5th Edition, 1989, Delmar Publishers Inc.)*

- ■Position other hand beside index finger (Figure C-8).
11. Place your shoulders over resident's sternum, keep your elbows straight. Interlace your fingers (Figure C-9) and begin compressions at the rate of 80-110 per minute (Figure C-10).
12. Compress 1-1/2 to 2 inches with equal compression and relaxation.
13. Maintain contact so landmark position is not lost.

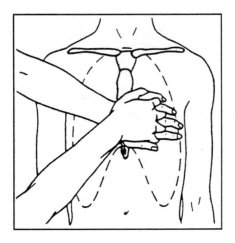

FIGURE C-9. Lace fingers of hands and keep them up off the chest. *(From Caldwell and Hegner,* Nursing Assistant, A Nursing Process Approach, *5th Edition, 1989, Delmar Publishers Inc.)*

14. Count out loud while completing 15 compressions and then do two ventilations.
15. Complete four cycles and then check for carotid pulse. If no pulse, ventilate two times and continue with compressions. Check carotid pulse every few minutes.

CPR (Two Person) (For Adult Victim)

1. If another person can assist, that person begins immediately after first rescuer completes a cycle of 15 compressions and two ventilations.

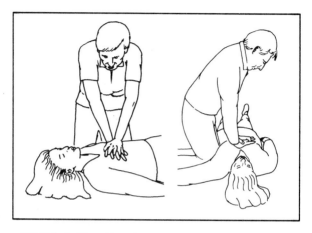

FIGURE C-10. Maintain this position while doing compressions at the rate of 80-110 per minute. *(From Caldwell and Hegner, Nursing Assistant, A Nursing Process Approach, 5th Edition, 1989, Delmar Publishers Inc.)*

2. Second rescuer moves to head.
   - ■Open airway with head-tilt/chin-lift method.
   - ■Check for carotid pulse.
3. First rescuer (compressor) finds landmark for proper hand position.
4. If no pulse, second rescuer (ventilator) gives one breath and compressor begins external chest compressions, counting one and, two and, three and, four and, five.
5. At completion of fifth compression, compressor pauses to allow ventilator to give one ventilation.

6. The ratio of five compressions to one ventilation is maintained, with carotid pulse checks every few minutes.
7. When rescuers switch positions, compressor gives a clear signal to change.
    - Compressor completes fifth compression.
    - Ventilator completes ventilation.
    - Ventilator moves to chest to become compressor and finds landmark for hand position.
    - Compressor moves to head to become ventilator and checks carotid pulse.
    - If no pulse, ventilator says, "no pulse," ventilates once, and the two rescuers resume CPR.

Obstructed Airway: Conscious Victim (Heimlich Maneuver)

1. If resident can cough or speak, do not interfere.
2. If resident cannot cough or speak, tell resident you are going to help her/him.
3. Stand behind resident and wrap your arms around resident's waist.
4. Make a fist with one hand, placing thumb side of fist against resident's abdomen, midway between navel and xiphoid process (Figure C-11).
5. Grasp your fist with your other hand and press fist into resident's abdomen with quick upward thrust.
6. Repeat thrusts until foreign body is expelled or resident loses consciousness.

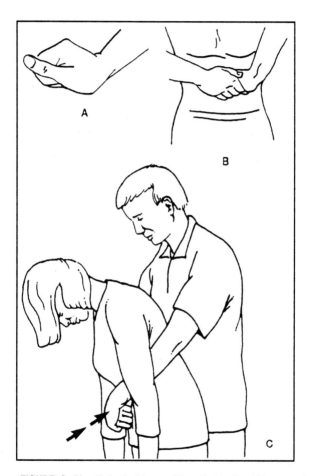

FIGURE C-11. Abdominal thrusts *(From Caldwell and Hegner, Nursing Assistant, A Nursing Process Approach, 5th Edition, 1989, Delmar Publishers Inc.)*

Obstructed Airway: Unconscious Victim

1. Place resident on back with face up and arms at sides.
2. Open resident's mouth with tongue-jaw lift method and sweep deeply into mouth to remove foreign body if possible.
3. If foreign body is not removed, open airway with head-tilt/chin-lift method. Seal mouth and nose. Attempt to ventilate.
4. Straddle resident's thighs. Place heel of one hand against resident's abdomen, midway

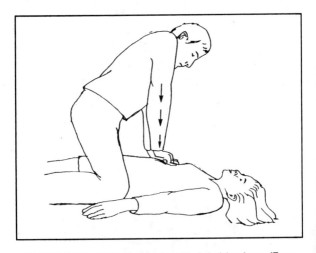

FIGURE C–12. Abdominal thrusts with victim lying down *(From Caldwell and Hegner,* Nursing Assistant, A Nursing Process Approach, *5th Edition, 1989, Delmar Publishers Inc.)*

between navel and xiphoid process (Figure C-12).

5. Place second hand on top of first hand and press into abdomen with quick, upward thrusts. Perform 6-10 thrusts.
6. If foreign body is still not expelled, repeat Steps 2-6 until successful.

3. GUIDELINES FOR OTHER EMERGENCIES

Fainting

1. If resident is ambulating, assist resident to floor to avoid injuries. Protect head and neck.
2. Help resident assume a protected position, sitting or lying down.
3. Loosen tight clothing.
4. Position head lower than heart to encourage cerebral blood flow.
5. Allow resident to rest for at least 10 minutes.
6. Maintain normal body temperature.
7. If resident has fallen, do not move resident until nurse has evaluated the situation.

Hemorrhage (External)

(NOTE: Gloves should be accessible throughout the facility. If there is time, put on gloves before coming into contact with blood. This is in accordance with universal precautions.)

1. Identify location of bleeding area.
2. Apply continuous, direct pressure over bleeding area with pad.

3. If seepage occurs, increase padding and pressure.
4. Keep resident warm and quiet until help arrives.

Hypoglycemia (Insulin Reaction, Low Blood Sugar)

(NOTE: Closely observe residents with diabetes. They may rapidly develop hypoglycemia, particularly if they take insulin. Immediate attention is required to prevent complications. Hypoglycemia may occur if the resident has not had sufficient food and fluid intake. (It can also occur if the resident has exercised more than usual.)

1. Signs and symptoms of hypoglycemia are:
   - Hunger.
   - Headache.
   - Dizziness and faintness.
   - Excessive perspiration, pale skin.
   - Trembling, nervousness, irritability, personality change.
   - Blurred vision.
   - Seizures and coma if allowed to continue.
   - Urine tests are negative for sugar. Blood sugar is low.
2. Immediate treatment:
   - Resident needs immediate carbohydrates such as orange juice, candy, jam, or syrup.
   - Know ahead of time what the procedure is in your facility.
   - Always know which residents are diabetic.

Hyperglycemia (High Blood Sugar, Diabetic Coma or Diabetic Acidosis)

(NOTE: This condition occurs when the amount of sugar in the blood is excessive. This can happen to residents with diabetes or to individuals who do not know they have diabetes.)

1. Signs and symptoms of hyperglycemia:
   - Dry, flushed, warm skin.
   - Nausea and/or vomiting.
   - Increased thirst.
   - Increased urination.
   - Fruity odor to the breath.
   - Aching.
   - Rapid, labored breathing.
   - Coma occurs if treatment is not given.
   - Urine and blood tests for sugar will show very large amounts of sugar.
2. Immediate treatment:
   - Resident is acutely ill; transfer to a hospital may be necessary, depending on policy of the facility.
   - IV feedings are usually initiated promptly.

Poisoning

(NOTE: If it is suspected that a resident has ingested a poisonous substance, immediately report to the nurse for instructions.)

Seizures

1. Do not leave resident alone.
2. Do not restrain movements.

3. Protect from injury. Move any objects that might cause injury.
4. Place small pillow, folded towel, or blanket under resident's head if resident is on floor.
5. Loosen clothing around head.
6. Maintain open airway.
7. Observe seizure.
8. After movements subside, turn resident on side so fluid or vomitus can drain freely.
9. Allow resident to rest.
10. Give mouth-to-mouth ventilations if breathing is not resumed following seizure.

Shock

1. Signs and symptoms of shock include:
   - Pale, cold, moist skin.
   - Complaints of feeling weak.
   - Weak, rapid pulse.
   - Increased and irregular breathing.
   - Restlessness and anxiety.
   - Perspiration.
2. Later signs of shock include:
   - Mottled skin.
   - Lack of response.
   - Sunken eyes with dilated pupils and vacant expression.
   - Loss of consciousness.
   - Drop in body temperature.
3. Immediate treatment:
   - Keep resident lying down and quiet.
   - Maintain normal body temperature.
   - Follow further instructions from nurse.

TABLE OF CONTENTS

SECTION D: INFECTION CONTROL

The prevention of complications is a major concern for employees in long-term care facilities. Infections are one complication that may be prevented by following these guidelines and your facility policies.

1. GENERAL GUIDELINES FOR PREVENTING INFECTIONS

1. Assist residents to maintain adequate fluid and food intake.
2. Assist residents to perform activity/exercise programs:
   - Follow positioning schedules.
   - Do passive range of motion exercises as ordered.
   - Remind/help residents to ambulate.
   - Encourage participation in exercise programs.
3. Attend to residents' personal hygiene needs promptly.
4. Toilet residents regularly to keep bladder empty.
5. Perform catheter care regularly and as directed. Avoid opening drainage system.
6. Observe residents carefully and report unusual signs:
   - Changes in urination.
     — Changes in frequency of urination or amount of urine voided.
     — Complaints of pain or burning upon urination.
     — Changes in character of urine.
   - Coughing or respiratory problems.

- ■ Confusion/disorientation that was not present before or that has increased.
- ■ Drainage or discharge from any body opening or skin wound.
- ■ Changes in skin color.
- ■ Complaints of pain, discomfort, or nausea.
- ■ Elevated temperature.
- ■ Red, swollen areas on body.

7. Remember to wash your hands before and after caring for a resident.
8. Disinfect all nondisposable equipment according to facility policy. Follow manufacturer's recommendations for using the disinfectant.

2. GUIDELINES FOR MEDICAL ASEPSIS

Medical asepsis means to maintain a state of cleanliness. Implementing the following principles prevents the spread of microorganisms between residents and staff.

1. Wash hands frequently and thoroughly.
2. Clean up dishes immediately after use.
3. Damp dust daily.
4. Provide bags for disposal of used tissues.
5. Turn face to one side to avoid breathing on resident.
6. Cover nose and mouth when coughing and sneezing.
7. Maintain good personal hygiene and grooming for self and for residents.

8. Immediately treat breaks in skin.
9. Disinfect or sterilize equipment used by more than one resident, after each use.
10. Maintain schedules for routine disinfection or sterilization of all equipment used for resident care.
11. Do not use personal care items for more than one resident.
12. Label all personal care items with residents' names.
13. Empty waste baskets frequently.
14. Follow facility policy for disposal of infectious waste.
15. Prevent blood and body fluids from splashing or spraying.
16. Avoid shaking bed linens.
17. Do not let dirty linens touch the floor.
18. Carry linens away from your uniform.
19. Empty linen inward with dirtiest area in center.
20. Do not eat food from residents' trays.

3. GUIDELINES FOR UNIVERSAL PRECAUTIONS

Universal precautions are implemented routinely in all health care facilities. This protects the health care provider from harmful microorganisms that may be transmitted from residents with undiagnosed infectious disease. The following guidelines are implemented with universal precautions.

1. Wear gloves for any contact with blood, body fluids, mucous membranes, or non-

intact skin. Change gloves after contact with each resident.

2. Wash hands immediately after gloves are removed. Wash hands and other skin surfaces immediately if contaminated with blood or other body fluids.

3. Wear impervious (water proof) gown or apron for procedures likely to generate splashes of blood or other body fluids.

4. Wear masks and protective eyewear for procedures likely to generate splashes of blood or other body fluids.

5. Dispose of needles with syringes and other sharp items in puncture-resistant container near point of use.

6. Do not recap needles or otherwise manipulate them by hand before disposal.

7. Mouthpieces or resuscitator bags should be available to minimize the need for emergency mouth-to-mouth resuscitation.

8. Waste and soiled linen should be handled according to facility policy for infectious waste disposal.

9. Immediately wipe up blood spills:
   - Use disposable gloves.
   - Use 1:10 dilution of bleach or disinfectant required by facility policy (Figure D-1).
   - Use disposable cleaning cloths.
   - Dispose of gloves and cleaning cloths in appropriate infectious waste receptacle.

(**NOTE:** See Section I, Procedures, for Isolation Procedures.)

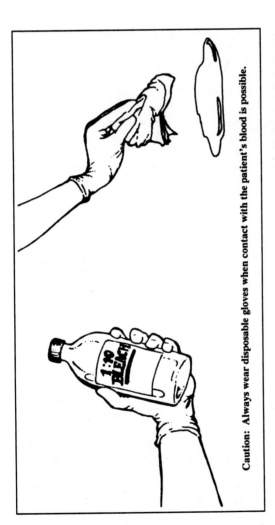

Caution: Always wear disposable gloves when contact with the patient's blood is possible.

FIGURE D-1 Immediately clean all blood spills with a 1:10 dilution of bleach or disinfectant, according to facility policy. *(From Caldwell and Hegner, Nursing Assistant, A Nursing Process Approach, 5th Edition, 1989, Delmar Publishers Inc.)*

4. GUIDELINES FOR STERILE PROCEDURES

In some facilities, nursing assistants are not expected to perform procedures requiring sterile techniques. If you are responsible for sterile procedures, you should be given thorough training before doing them.

Sterile Gloves, Opening

To open a package of sterile gloves without contaminating the gloves:

1. Wash your hands.
2. Assemble equipment:
   - Sterile gloves in correct size
3. Gloves are arranged in package so when it is opened, they are on proper side for gloving.
   - Palms are up with thumbs pointing to outer edge.
   - Wrists are cuffed and folded over.
4. The inside only of the glove comes in contact with the skin. If the outside of the glove is touched, it is considered contaminated and cannot be used for any sterile procedure.
5. When putting on gloves, remember that glove surfaces touch only sterile items.
6. Procedure completion actions:
   - Dispose of glove wrapper.
   - Dispose of soiled gloves when finished.

Sterile Package, Opening

To open sterile package without contaminating the contents:

1. Wash your hands.
2. Assemble equipment:
   ■ Sterile package
   ■ Sterile transfer forceps if needed
3. Most packages have a seal that changes color to indicate the sterilizing process has been completed.
4. If color code has not changed or seal does not look intact, do not consider article sterile. *If you have any doubt about sterility, consider item unsterile.*
5. Touch only outside of package. Only sterile surfaces contact other sterile surfaces.
6. Commercially prepared products will be sealed. If package is in poor condition or discolored, do not consider item sterile. Discard item.
7. Transfer forceps are instruments used to pick up sterile items. They are lifted by the handle, being careful not to touch sterile tips to anything not sterile.

TABLE OF CONTENTS

SECTION E: COMMUNICATIONS

The process of communication involves the exchange of information. As a nursing assistant, you can facilitate this process by using effective methods of communication with other employees. You can do much to increase the quality of life for residents in your facility by appropriately communicating with each resident. Follow these guidelines when communicating with coworkers or residents.

1. GENERAL GUIDELINES FOR COMMUNICATION

Verbal Communication (Spoken)

When communicating verbally with others, be aware of:

1. Tone of voice.
2. Voice loudness.
3. Articulation.
4. Words or phrases with double meanings, or cultural meanings that could be misunderstood.
5. Swearing or using slang.

Nonverbal Communication

Your body language can sometimes speak louder than words. Be aware of the message that is being sent through:

1. Body posture.
2. Body position.

3. Hand and body movements.
4. Facial expressions.
5. Activity level.
6. Overall appearance.

2. GUIDELINES FOR STAFF COMMUNICATION

Staff members communicate with each other in several different ways.

Shift Report

1. Listen for name and location of your assigned residents.
2. Residents' diagnoses and physicians' names.
3. Special instructions for residents' care.
4. Incidents, unusual situations, acute illnesses, or changes in condition during the last 24 hours.

Giving Report to Nurse

1. Give name and location of your assigned residents.
2. Discuss care that was given.
3. Report care that was not given and the reason why it was not given.
4. Report observations.
5. Report residents' reactions and comments.

Answering Telephone

1. Identify unit.

2. Identify yourself and your position, for example, "Mary Smith, CNA."
3. Ask caller's name then ask caller to wait while you get the person called.
4. If person is unavailable, take a message:
   - Date.
   - Time.
   - Caller's name and telephone number.
   - Write message clearly.
   - Sign message with your name and title, such as "Mary Smith, CNA."

(**NOTE:** Be sure you know how to use the telephone system correctly. Be careful when transferring calls so you do not cut off the caller.)

Documentation (See Section H, Observing and Reporting)

Care-plan Conference

The care-plan conference provides the interdisciplinary team with the opportunity to evaluate residents' conditions and problems. The team members develop possible solutions to problems by establishing approaches or interventions and setting goals. The family and resident are team members. As a nursing assistant you are also a valuable team member.

1. Provide information about resident concerning:
   - New problems.
   - Progress in meeting goals for previous

        problems.
- ■ Effectiveness of approaches or interventions being used to help residents meet goals.
2. Present ideas for:
   - ■ Resolving new problems.
   - ■ New approaches to old problems that are not being resolved.
3. Listen to ideas and information presented by other team members.

Inservice Programs

Inservice programs are a method for communicating information to staff members. This information may pertain to:

1. New policies being implemented by the facility.
2. New procedures involving resident care.
3. Use of new equipment.
4. Caring for a resident with an unusual diagnosis or unique problems.
5. Results of studies/research done within the facility.
6. Issues in health care.
7. Problem solving for nonresident issues.

3. GUIDELINES FOR COMMUNICATING WITH RESIDENTS

1. Be sure you have residents' attention.
2. Use nonthreatening words or gestures.

3. Speak clearly and courteously.
4. Use a pleasant tone of voice.
5. Use appropriate body language.
6. Be alert to residents' needs to communicate with you. Allow time for residents to talk and respond. Show interest and concern.
7. Do not speak about residents in front of other residents.
8. Do not interrupt residents.
9. Reflect residents' feelings and thoughts by rewording residents' statements into questions.
10. Ask for clarification if you are unsure of what residents are saying.
11. Give residents only factual information, not your personal feelings, opinions, or beliefs.
12. Information concerning residents' condition, medications, and treatments should be given by the physician or nurse.
13. Do not argue with residents.

4. GUIDELINES FOR COMMUNICATING WITH RESIDENTS WITH SPECIAL NEEDS

(NOTE: Always check the care plan before attempting to communicate with a resident with special communication needs. Specific approaches may be established for all staff members to use with the resident.

Lack of consistency in using these approaches is confusing and frustrating to the resident.)

Communicating with Hearing Impaired Residents

1. First get resident's attention.
   - ■ Make sure the resident sees you.
   - ■ Touch resident lightly to indicate you wish to speak.
2. If resident uses a hearing aid, be sure resident is wearing it and that hearing aid is on.
3. If resident has a "good" ear, stand or sit on that side.
4. Don't chew gum, eat, or cover your mouth while talking.
5. Light should be behind the resident so your face can be clearly seen.
6. Face the resident; many hearing impaired people can read lips or interpret your facial expressions.
7. Reduce outside distractions. Speak in a quiet, calm manner.
8. Start conversation with a key word or phrase so resident has clues as to what you are saying.
9. Keep your voice pitch low.
10. Speak slowly, distinctly, and naturally.
11. Form words carefully, use familiar words, and keep sentences short.
12. Rephrase words as needed.

13. Shouting, mouthing or exaggerating words, or speaking very slowly only make it harder for resident to understand you.

14. Use facial expressions, gestures, and body language to help express your meanings.

15. Some hearing impaired residents use sign language.
    - Signing depends on hand and finger movements and facial expressions.
    - This is a skill that requires learning and practice.
    - There are different forms of sign language just as there are different spoken languages.
    - There are some basic signs that may be helpful (Figure E-1).

16. Residents who have been hearing impaired for several years may have speech that is difficult to understand.

17. Some hearing impaired people are embarrassed to tell you when they do not understand you.

18. People who cannot hear may appear confused when they are not.

Communicating with Visually Impaired Residents

1. When approaching a visually impaired person, address person by name and then lightly touch hand or arm to avoid startling.

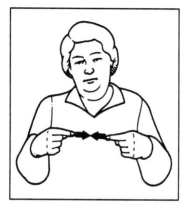

A. Hurt, Pain, Ache, Sore. Palms face chest and index fingers extend toward one another but do not touch. Thrust hands toward each other several times to indicate hurt, pain, ache, or sore.

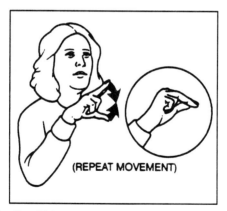

(REPEAT MOVEMENT)

B. No. Extend index and middle fingers, bringing them down to meet thumb in two quick movements for the word "no."

FIGURE E-1 Signing *(From Caldwell and Hegner,* Nursing Assistant, A Nursing Process Approach, *5th Edition, 1989, Delmar Publishers Inc.)*

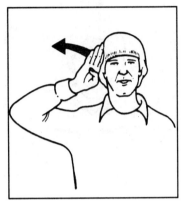

C. Hello or Hi. Start with index finger of right hand at right temple with palm forward and fingers pointing up. Bring hand outward to the right to express "hello" or "hi."

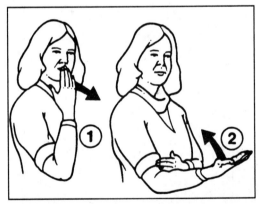

D. Good Morning. Start with fingertips of right open hand toward face. Touch lips and bring hand down, bending elbow. Touch inner elbow with left open hand as right hand is brought upward to express "good morning."

FIGURE E-1 Signing (continued)

2. After you speak to resident, identify yourself and explain why you are there. For example, "Hello, Mr. Smith. My name is Mary Jones, and I would like to take your blood pressure."

3. Be specific when giving directions. For example, "I am putting your mail on the right side of your bedside stand."

4. When giving directions to locate an area in the building, tell resident how many doors will be passed and when he/she should turn right or left.

5. When you leave the resident, make sure you announce your departure. For example, "I am leaving your room now. Can I get you anything else?"

6. Offer to read mail to visually impaired residents.

7. If resident has a telephone, make sure he/she can use it. (Resident can count numbers on dial to make calls.)

8. Tactfully inform visually impaired resident if clothing is soiled, unmatched, or in need of repair.

9. Encourage resident to listen to radio or TV to keep up with news and current events.

10. Make sure resident is aware of talking book machines. Inform social services department if resident wishes to use these.

11. Describe environment and objects around resident so a frame of reference is developed. This helps avoid disorientation related to vision impairment.

Communicating with Residents with Aphasia

1. Face resident and make eye contact before speaking.

2. Say resident's name and give a social greeting before asking questions or giving instructions.

3. Speak slowly and clearly. Use short, complete sentences.

4. Pause between sentences to allow resident time to comprehend and interpret what you said.

5. Check resident's comprehension before you proceed. Ask a question based on information you just gave the resident.

6. Use nonverbal cues to augment spoken communication. Use gestures, facial expressions, or pictures.

7. Ask questions that require only short responses or ones that can be answered nonverbally.

8. Repeat what resident just said to help resident keep focused on the conversation.

9. Find out if the speech therapist has devised methods of nonverbal communication, such as communication boards or picture books.

10. Do not avoid talking to a person with aphasia. Do not shout to try and make him/her understand.

11. If you sense frustration, let resident know you are aware of the frustration. Suggest that you talk about something else and then try again.

Communicating with Residents with Dementia

1. Begin conversation by identifying yourself and calling resident by name. Do not ask if resident remembers you or knows who you are.
2. Talk to resident at eye level and maintain eye contact.
3. Maintain a pleasant facial expression while you are talking and listening.
4. Place a hand on resident's arm or hand unless this causes agitation.
5. Make sure resident can hear you. Avoid distractions of noise and activity.
6. Use a lower tone of voice.
7. Use short, common words and short, simple sentences.
8. Give resident time to respond.
9. Ask only one simple question at a time. If you must repeat it, say it exactly the same way.
10. Ask resident to do only one task at a time.
11. Residents with dementia will eventually be unable to comprehend verbal communication.
    - Use pictures, point, touch, or hand resident items.
    - Demonstrate an action when you want resident to complete a task.
12. The resident may use word substitutes. If these are consistent, find out what they mean. Use them yourself to see if resident understands you better.

13. Avoid abstract, common expressions. For example, "You can hop into bed now," means just that to the resident.
14. Repeat resident's last words to help him/her stay on track during conversation.
15. Do not try to "make" resident understand. Avoid lengthy explanations and excessive verbal communication. This tends to agitate most people with dementia.
16. Use nonverbal praise freely and always respect feelings.

Psychosocial Support

TABLE OF CONTENTS

SECTION F: PSYCHOSOCIAL SUPPORT

---

1. GENERAL GUIDELINES FOR PROVIDING PSYCHOSOCIAL SUPPORT

1. As a nursing assistant, you can do much to help residents meet their needs while they are living in the long-term care facility.

2. Remember that emotional needs cannot be fulfilled unless the residents' physical and safety needs are first met.

3. All people have a need to (Figure F–1):
   - Love and be loved.
   - Feel respect from others.
   - Feel that self-esteem is protected.

4. Many residents are adjusting to changes of aging:
   - Decreased physical strength.
   - Retirement and reduced income.
   - Death of a spouse and other loved ones.
   - A need to tie up "loose ends" in preparation for dying.

5. Newer residents are also adjusting to living in the long-term care facility:
   - Developing trust in staff members.
   - Becoming acquainted with other residents.
   - Adapting to routine of the facility.
   - Having less personal space.
   - Giving up a home and furnishings.
   - Relinquishing unfulfilled dreams for the future.
   - Giving up favorite activities because of impaired abilities.

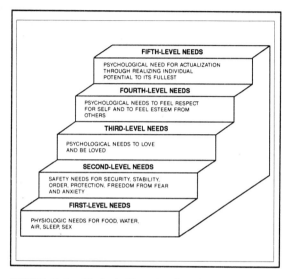

FIGURE F-1 Maslow's hierarchy of needs is the same for people of all ages. *(From Caldwell and Hegner, Nursing Assistant, A Nursing Process Approach, 5th Edition, 1989, Delmar Publishers Inc.)*

- Coping with discomfort associated with health problems.
- Having to depend on others for meeting physical needs if resident is permanently or temporarily disabled.
- Coping with disrupted personal relationships.

6. You can assist residents to make adjustments by:

- Respecting all the residents' rights.
- Keeping information confidential.
- Listening carefully to everything residents say.
- Recognizing that each resident is an individual with likes and dislikes.
- Answering signal lights promptly.
- Treating all residents as adults.
- Understanding that it takes time for residents and families to adjust to long-term care admission.
- Assisting residents to maintain spiritual/religious practices and beliefs.
- Reporting signs of physical discomfort or mental anxiety to the nurse so steps can be taken to resolve problems.

7. Help residents feel loved and accepted by:
   - Accepting each resident in a nonjudgmental manner.
   - Use touch appropriately to indicate your acceptance of the person.
   - Provide privacy when family and friends visit.
   - Encourage residents to participate in facility activities.
   - Assist residents to meet other residents.
   - Give sincere compliments to residents.
   - Respect and understand the lifelong need for sexuality.
   - Show you care with your verbal and nonverbal communications.

8. Help residents feel self-esteem and respect from others:

■ Help residents maintain an identity by:
  — Calling them by the names/titles of their choice.
  — Learning about them, their families, and their histories.
  — Helping them with their choice of hairstyles, clothing, use of makeup and jewelry.
  — Encouraging them to use their personal possessions to personalize their rooms.
■ Give residents as many choices as possible.
■ Respect their decisions.
■ Respect their privacy and space by:
  — Allowing them to arrange their rooms as they desire unless this interferes with health or safety.
  — Showing respect for all their belongings.
■ Help residents feel useful by asking for their help. Unless they choose not to, they might:
  — Deliver mail to other residents.
  — Stuff envelopes for mailings.
  — Care for nursing home pets, such as birds or fish.
  — Serve as officers on Residents' Council.
  — Play the piano or lead singing groups.
  — Lead current event groups.
  — Knit or crochet items for gift shop.
  — Contribute articles, jokes, or drawings for the facility newsletter.

■ Encourage independence to the extent possible.
— Avoid forcing dependence by doing ADL's for residents who can do them alone.
— Give praise.

Using Defense Mechanisms

When needs go unfulfilled or the ability to cope with stress is diminished, residents may use defense mechanisms to protect their self-esteem. Recognize residents' needs to use defense mechanisms. These are harmful only when they become the major way of dealing with stressful situations. If this occurs, an experienced mental health professional may provide counseling for the resident. Here are some definitions for common defense mechanisms.

1. Repression
   ■ Unconsciously refusing to recognize a painful thought, memory, feeling, or impulse.
2. Suppression
   ■ Deliberately (consciously) refusing to recognize a painful thought, memory, feeling, or impulse.
3. Projection
   ■ Attributing one's own unacceptable feelings and thoughts to others.
4. Denial
   ■ Blocking out painful or anxiety-producing events or feelings.

5. Reaction formation
   - ■ Repressing the reality of a situation and then exhibiting behaviors that are the opposite of the real feelings.

To Assist Residents to Cope

1. Be a good listener.
2. Be sensitive to nonverbal messages that may give clues to source of stress.
3. Treat person with respect, recognizing him/her as a unique individual.
4. Never label residents' behavior and use the label in describing residents.
5. Let residents know by your actions you are dependable and trustworthy.
6. Do not argue or enter into a power struggle with a resident, even when you know resident is wrong.
7. Try to determine source of stress and find a way to reduce it.
8. Be supportive of person's own attempts to overcome the stress.

Unusual Behaviors

Residents who display unusual behaviors are usually reacting to a situation in which they are not able to meet their psychosocial needs. They are frustrated by their lack of control and resort to these behaviors in an attempt to satisfy unfilled needs and to ease anxieties. Here are some guidelines for caring for residents with these behaviors.

1. Demanding behavior
   - Try to learn and appreciate factors that are causing the behavior.
   - Listen to residents and be sensitive to body language.
   - Be consistent in caregiving so residents feel secure.
   - Do not take demands personally.
   - Make attempts to provide care before residents have to "demand" it.
2. Manipulative behavior
   - If resident with manipulative behavior compliments you, accept compliment graciously and matter of factly. Do not allow compliments to influence your judgment or cause you to show favoritism to the resident.
   - Residents with manipulative behaviors may voice criticisms of other staff members to you. Avoid agreeing with critical comments. If resident persists in the comments, tactfully tell her/him that she/he will have to talk to the nurse or social worker about the problems.
   - Do not falsely label a resident as manipulative. Compliments may be sincere and resident may have real problems with another staff member. Relay concerns to nurse or social worker if the behavior becomes a pattern.
   - All staff members should treat residents in a consistent manner.

■Develop a sense of trust with residents. Don't make promises you can't keep. Honor requests promptly.

2. GUIDELINES FOR ASSISTING RESIDENTS EXHIBITING MALADAPTIVE BEHAVIORS

Maladaptive behaviors may be noted when a resident is unable to function smoothly with staff, other residents and perhaps family. These situations require assessment and planning by members of the interdisciplinary team. Interventions by a mental health professional or psychiatrist are often necessary. You can help residents with these behaviors in the following ways:

Depression

1. Stress resident's worth and assist resident in using available support systems.
2. Do not pity resident. This validates depressed feelings.
3. Make sure resident has eyeglasses and hearing aids if these are needed.
4. Provide resident with activities that help resident think beyond self.
5. Avoid tiring activities.
6. Use simple language and speak more slowly.
7. Encourage and assist resident to participate in activities involving physical exercise.

8. Monitor intake, elimination, and sleep patterns. Depression may cause major changes in these functions.

Be alert for potential suicide. Watch for and report:

9. A change in response or mood.
10. Withdrawal or secretiveness.
11. Sudden loss of a support system.
12. Refusal of food, fluids, care, or medications.
13. Sudden interest or disinterest in religion.
14. Attempts to obtain scissors, knives, or other dangerous objects.
15. Statements about "ending it all," "killing myself," "nothing to live for."
16. An inability to complete simple tasks without a physical reason.
17. Deep preoccupation with something that cannot be explained.

Disorientation

Disorientation may be permanent because of Alzheimer's Disease or other dementias. The disorientation cannot be reversed in these situations. Disorientation may be temporary due to environmental changes, acute illness, or stressful situations. When this is the case, disorientation will diminish when the underlying cause is treated. In all cases:

1. Be calm and gentle.
2. Be consistent in your care and in your approach to the resident.

3. Provide resident with a structured but flexible routine.
4. Maintain a peaceful, quiet, simple, uncluttered, and unchanging environment.
5. Avoid trying to "reason" with or to make resident "understand" what he/she is not capable of understanding.
6. Watch for facial expressions and body language for clues to feelings and moods.
7. Learn what triggers agitation and anger and work to prevent these situations.
8. Attend to resident's physical needs promptly.
9. Avoid using restraints.
10. Use reality orientation appropriately.
11. Allow resident to do what he/she is capable of doing.
12. Use touch appropriately.
13. Watch your body language and be sensitive to resident's response.
14. Do not "crowd" resident by being too close or having too many people around him/her.
15. Always treat the resident as a worthy, dignified adult.

TABLE OF CONTENTS

SECTION G: ABBREVIATIONS

1. BODY PARTS

abd	–	abdomen
bld	–	blood
BK	–	below the knee
CNS	–	central nervous system
G.B.	–	gallbladder
G.I.	–	gastrointestinal
G.U.	–	genitourinary
H&L	–	heart and lungs
jt	–	joint
lt	–	left
O.D.	–	right eye
O.S.	–	left eye
os	–	mouth
O.U.	–	both eyes
vag	–	vagina, vaginal

2. DIAGNOSIS

AFB	–	acid fast bacillus
AIDS	–	acquired immune deficiency syndrome
AKA	–	above the knee amputation
ARC	–	AIDS related complex
ASHD	–	arteriosclerotic heart disease
AD	–	Alzheimer's Disease
BPH	–	benign prostatic hypertrophy
CA	–	cancer
CAD	–	coronary artery disease
CHD	–	coronary heart disease
CHF	–	congestive heart failure
CVA	–	cerebral vascular accident; stroke

DOA	–	dead on arrival
DM	–	diabetes mellitus
FB	–	foreign body
FUO	–	fever of unknown origin
Fx	–	fracture
IH	–	infectious hepatitis
KA	–	Kaposi's sarcoma
LBP	–	low back pain
MI	–	myocardial infarction
MS	–	multiple sclerosis
OBS	–	organic brain syndrome
PD	–	Parkinson's Disease
PVD	–	peripheral vascular disease
RA	–	rheumatoid arthritis
RHD	–	rheumatic heart disease
SDAT	–	senile dementia of Alzheimer's type
TIA	–	transient ischemic attack
TUR	–	transurethral resection
URI	–	upper respiratory infection
UTI	–	urinary tract infection

3. RESIDENT ORDERS AND CHARTING

aa	–	of each
ADL	–	activities of daily living
ad lib	–	as desired
adm	–	admission
amb	–	ambulatory
AMA	–	against medical advice
ASA	–	aspirin

ASAP	–	as soon as possible
as tol	–	as tolerated
B.M.	–	bowel movement
B/P	–	blood pressure
B.R.	–	bedrest
BRP	–	bathroom privileges
c̄	–	with
cath	–	catheterize
CBR	–	complete bedrest
ck	–	check
cl liq	–	clear liquid
DAT	–	diet as tolerated
DC, D/C	–	discontinue
disch	–	discharge
DNR	–	do not resuscitate
Dr.	–	doctor
drsg	–	dressing
D/S	–	dextrose and saline
DSD	–	dry, sterile dressing
DW	–	distilled water
D/W	–	dextrose and water
Dx	–	diagnosis
et	–	and
HOB	–	head of bed
irrig	–	irrigation
isol	–	isolation
I.V.	–	intravenous
KO	–	keep open
lap	–	laparotomy
lg	–	large
liq	–	liquid

LPM	–	liters per minute
max	–	maximum
min	–	minimum
mod	–	moderate
Na	–	sodium
N/C	–	no complaints
neg	–	negative
NG	–	nasogastric
N.P.O.	–	nothing by mouth
N/S	–	normal saline
N&V	–	nausea and vomiting
NVD	–	nausea, vomiting, diarrhea
O2	–	oxygen
OOB	–	out of bed
per	–	by
pH	–	acidity
p.o.	–	by mouth
prep	–	prepare
p.r.n.	–	whenever necessary
prom	–	passive range of motion
q.s.	–	quantity sufficient
rehab	–	rehabilitation
resp	–	respiration
rom	–	range of motion
rt	–	right or routine
Rx	–	treatment
$\bar{s}$	–	without
semi	–	half
sm	–	small
$\overline{ss}$	–	one half
sos	–	if necessary

spec	–	specimen
SSE	–	soapsuds enema
stat	–	at once
Surg	–	surgery
TPN	–	total parenteral nutrition
TWE	–	tap water enema
Tx	–	traction
ur	–	urine
w/c	–	wheelchair

4. PHYSICAL AND HISTORY

DOB	–	date of birth
FH	–	family history
Hx	–	history
LMP	–	last menstrual period
L&W	–	living and well
M&F	–	mother and father
MH	–	marital history
PE	–	physical exam
PI	–	present illness
PMH	–	past medical history
Px	–	prognosis
R/O	–	rule out
Sx	–	symptom
UCD	–	usual childhood diseases
UK	–	unknown
WDWN	–	well-developed, well-nourished
YOB	–	year of birth

5. TESTS

ABC	–	aspiration, biopsy, cytology
ABG	–	arterial blood gas study
CBC	–	complete blood count
EEG	–	electroencephalogram
EKG, ECG	–	electrocardiogram
FBS	–	fasting blood sugar
GA	–	gastric analysis
Hb	–	hemoglobin
HCT	–	hematocrit
MRI	–	magnetic resonance imaging
myel	–	myelogram
PPD	–	purified protein derivative
RBC	–	red blood count
S&A	–	sugar and acetone
UA	–	urinalysis
WBC	–	white blood count

6. PLACES OR DEPARTMENTS

ACT	–	activities
CS	–	central supply
ES	–	environmental services
Nrsg	–	nursing
OT	–	occupational therapy
PT	–	physical therapy
RT	–	respiratory therapy
ST	–	speech therapy
SS	–	social services

7. TIME

a.c.	–	before meals
A.M.	–	morning
b.i.d.	–	twice a day
BIN	–	twice a night
h	–	hour
h.s.	–	hour of sleep, bedtime
noc, noct	–	night
p	–	after
p.c.	–	after meals
P.M.	–	evening or afternoon
q	–	every
qd	–	every day
qh	–	every hour
q2h	–	every two hours
q.i.d.	–	four times a day
qm	–	every morning
qn	–	every night
qod	–	every other day
t.i.d.	–	three times a day
WA	–	while awake

8. ROMAN NUMERALS

I	–	1
II	–	2
III	–	3
IV	–	4
V	–	5
VI	–	6
VII	–	7
VIII	–	8
IX	–	9
X	–	10

9. MEASUREMENTS AND VOLUME

amt	–	amount
cc	–	cubic centimeter
dr	–	dram
gtt	–	drop
L	–	liter
ml	–	milliliter
oz	–	ounce
TBS	–	tablespoon
tsp	–	teaspoon

10. WEIGHT/HEIGHT

cm	–	centimeter
ht	–	height
in	–	inch
kg	–	kilogram
lb	–	pound
mm	–	millimeter
wt	–	weight

11. TEMPERATURE

ax	–	axillary
C	–	Celsius
°	–	degree
F	–	Fahrenheit
O	–	oral
R	–	rectal

TABLE OF CONTENTS

SECTION H: OBSERVING AND REPORTING

1. GENERAL GUIDELINES FOR MAKING OBSERVATIONS

1. Observations are made through the use of your senses.
   - Important information about the resident is noted through what you see and hear.
   - Your sense of smell and touch are also used to pick up unusual signs and symptoms.
2. Information is sometimes obtained by using equipment such as thermometers, scales, blood pressure cuffs, and stethoscopes.
3. Doing special procedures, such as urine testing, also provides information about the residents' conditions.
4. Establish a routine for making observations.
5. Keep in mind the age, sex, and known problems of residents when you make observations.
6. Get to know your residents so you immediately recognize changes.
7. Listen to what residents tell you.
8. Report unusual signs and symptoms to nurse.

2. GUIDELINES FOR PHYSICAL OBSERVATIONS

Think of the resident as a whole person instead of dwelling only on the known deviations of the individual. Systematically note the appearance and functional ability of the resident. Think of the possibilities outside the usual for that individual and note the presence or absence of these possibilities. These observations give information about the resident's body systems. Remember that some residents are unaware of changes that may be affecting their health. It is important that changes are noted and acted upon promptly.

1. Eyes
   - Drainage from any opening.
   - Eyes inflamed or crusting around eyelids.
   - Able to see with both eyes.
   - Complaints of blurring, clouding, rings around lights, spots, flashes.
   - Glasses or contact lenses required.

2. Ears
   - Drainage or excess wax in ears.
   - Outer ear inflamed.
   - Able to hear with both ears.
   - Complaints of ringing in ears.
   - Hearing aid required.

3. Nose
   - Nasal drainage or discharge.
   - Nose inflamed.
   - Able to smell odors.
   - Common odors smell unusual.

4. Mouth
   - Lips cracked, dry, swollen.
   - Tongue unusual color, white spots.
   - Sores noted anywhere in mouth.
   - Gums swollen, bleeding.
   - Teeth missing, discolored, broken.
   - Unusual odor from mouth.
   - Presence of dentures.

     ■ Able to taste foods and liquids.
     ■ Foods and liquids have unusual tastes.

5. Speech
     ■ Uses words appropriately (in context).
     ■ Slurred.
     ■ Mumbling.
     ■ Moderate voice tone.

6. Facial expression
     ■ Appropriate to the situation.
     ■ Facial expression is fixed, unchanging.
     ■ Both sides of face are involved in expressions.
     ■ Mouth is the same on both sides.

7. Hair and scalp
     ■ Dry.
     ■ Oily.
     ■ Fine.
     ■ Coarse.
     ■ Brittle.
     ■ Excessive loss of hair/bald spots.
     ■ Flaky scalp.

8. Skin
     ■ Color
        — Flushed
        — Pale
        — Cyanotic (dusky, bluish color)
        — Jaundiced (yellow/orange color)
     ■ Temperature and moistness
        — Hot
        — Warm
        — Cool
        — Dry, scaly
        — Damp/moist

■ Sense of touch
  — Can feel pressure, pain
  — Can feel hot, cold
  — Complaints of numbness, tingling
  — Excessive perspiration present
■ Integrity **(NOTE:** Be sure to check in all skin folds and pressure areas.)
  — Pressure areas/redness/skin broken/ drainage
  — Bruises, abrasions
  — Skin tears
  — Rashes
  — Change in moles
  — Areas of swelling, bumps, lumps
  — Scars

9. Extremities
   ■ Edema of hands/feet.
   ■ Nails
     — Cracked, chipped
     — Bloody
     — Dusky, pale color

10. Trunk/chest
    ■ Unusual shape.
    ■ Curvature or hump on back.
    ■ Unusual breathing patterns.
    ■ Breasts
      — Size, shape
      — Condition, appearance of nipples
      — Presence of discharge, lumps

11. Abdomen, pelvic and genital area
    ■ Abdomen soft, hard.
    ■ Discharge/drainage from penis, vagina.

12. Heart and lungs

- ■ Pulse
  - — Strong/bounding/weak/barely perceptible
  - — Regular/irregular
  - — Rate
- ■ Blood pressure.
- ■ Respirations
  - — Noisy (wheezing, rattling, gurgling)
  - — Difficult, labored (dyspnea)
  - — Periods of apnea
  - — Dry or productive coughing. If sputum is present, note amount, color.
  - — Shortness of breath with exertion

13. Gastrointestinal tract
    - ■ Appetite.
    - ■ Ability to chew, swallow.
    - ■ Complaints of nausea.
    - ■ Vomiting
      - — amount
      - — description
    - ■ Belching, burping.
    - ■ Expelling flatus.
    - ■ Bowel movements
      - — Frequency
      - — Amount
      - — Color
      - — Consistency
      - — Unusual odor
    - ■ Incontinent of bowels.

14. Urinary tract
    - ■ Urinary elimination
      - — Frequency
      - — Amount

— Color
— Clarity
— Unusual odor
■ Incontinent of urine.

15. Mental status
    ■ Difficult to arouse.
    ■ Dozes frequently.
    ■ Restless/pacing/wandering.
    ■ Withdrawn.
    ■ Angers easily.
    ■ Responds to own name; recognizes and identifies members of family; knows time and place.
    ■ Answers common questions correctly.
    ■ Makes simple decisions.
    ■ Follows instructions.

16. Pain/discomfort
    ■ Location of pain.
    ■ Pain starts in one location and then spreads to another area.
    ■ Duration of pain.
    ■ Pain changes in relation to body position or movement.
    ■ Pain comes and goes.
    ■ Resident had pain medication but pain is not subsiding.
    ■ Description of pain
      — Sharp
      — Dull
      — Burning
      — Aching
      — Knifelike

3. GUIDELINES FOR OBSERVATIONS FOR ACTIVITIES OF DAILY LIVING

These observations provide information on the resident's ability to perform activities of daily living. The resident's ability may change because of changes in strength, endurance, or extent of range of motion. Note any of the following changes.

1. Movement and activity
   - Range of motion during passive range of motion exercises is decreasing.
   - Movements rigid.
   - Tremors, wringing, or clenching of hands.
   - Presence of spasticity, contractures.
   - Note ability to
     — Sit upright without leaning, falling over.
     — Move self in bed.
     — Come to sitting position on edge of bed.
     — Move self in chair.
     — Propel own wheelchair.
     — Come to standing position.
   - Observe gait (walking) for:
     — Rigidity
     — Shuffling
     — Feet dragging
     — Limping
     — Stumbling easily
     — Losing balance
     — Use of assistive device: cane or walker
     — Use of leg/ankle/foot braces

2. Toileting. Note if resident:
   ■ Toilets self.
   ■ Manipulates clothing.
   ■ Cleans self after toileting.
   ■ Is continent of stool.
3. Bathing, grooming, hygiene. Note if resident
   ■ Holds items for bathing, grooming, hygiene (washcloth, comb, toothbrush, for example).
   ■ Uses these items correctly.
4. Eating. Note if resident:
   ■ Holds eating utensils correctly.
   ■ Uses eating utensils correctly.
   ■ Feeds self appropriately.

4. GUIDELINES FOR OBSERVATIONS OF RESIDENTS RECEIVING SPECIAL CARE PROCEDURES

Residents may require feeding tubes, intravenous feedings, or oxygen. These procedures are performed by the nurse or physician. Your responsibility as a nursing assistant is to observe the resident. Report any problems you note with the treatment or unusual reactions of the resident. These residents receive the same personal care as other residents.

Feeding Tubes

1. Feeding tube may be inserted:
   ■ Through nose, esophagus, and into stomach. This is called a nasogastric or N/G tube.

■Directly into stomach through an incision in abdominal wall. This is called a gastrostomy tube, or G tube.
■Directly into small intestines. This is called a jejunostomy tube or J tube.

(NOTE: Feeding tube may be connected to a pump. If alarm sounds, report to the nurse.)

2. Keep head of bed elevated at 30–40 degree angle during feeding and for 30 minutes afterward.
3. Check taping and dressings where tube is inserted. Report to nurse if they are loose.
4. Check tubing for kinks. Be sure it is not stretched and that resident is not lying on it.
5. Report to nurse if resident has retching, nausea, or vomiting.
6. Make sure end of tube is closed between feedings.
7. Note condition of resident's mouth when giving oral care. Oral care is needed more frequently.
8. Report to nurse if resident has loose stools.

Intravenous Feedings

Intravenous feedings (IVs) may be given because resident is dehydrated and requires fluids; medication needs to be administered in the vein; and resident requires additional nutrients. Make these observations as you care for the resident. Report the following changes to the nurse.

1. Flow rate changes or stops.
2. Drip chamber is full.
3. Make sure bag/bottle is always higher than infusion site.
4. Signs of redness, swelling, or pain at infusion site.
5. Infusion site is leaking.
6. Tubing is twisted, stretched, or disconnected from bottle or needle.

(**NOTE:** Make sure bag/bottle is always higher than infusion site.)

Oxygen

Residents with heart or lung disease may need oxygen. This can be administered by tent, nasal cannula, nasal catheter, or mask. Note the following items and report to the nurse if necessary.

1. No smoking is allowed in the area.
2. No-smoking and oxygen-in-use cards are posted on door and over bed.
3. Smoking materials have been removed from the room.
4. Cotton blankets are being used instead of wool blankets.
5. Resident is using handbell instead of electric signal cord.
6. Unneeded electrical equipment has been removed from the room.
7. Note flow rate.
8. If tank is used as oxygen source, be sure that:
   ■ There is sufficient oxygen (Figure H-1).

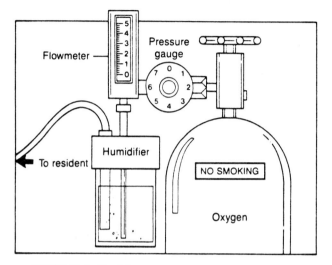

FIGURE H-1 Check flowmeter and gauge whenever resident is receiving oxygen. *(From Caldwell and Hegner,* Nursing Assistant, A Nursing Process Approach, *5th Edition, 1989, Delmar Publishers Inc.)*

- ■ Empty tanks are marked and returned to proper source for refilling.
- ■ Tank is secure and cannot fall.
9. Be sure there are no kinks in tubing.
10. Check humidifier jar and report if water is below fill line.
11. Oxygen tents
    - ■ Check plastic canopy for leaks.
    - ■ Canopy is tucked under mattress and secured across front of bed.
    - ■ Canopy zippers are closed unless care is being given.

12. Oxygen mask
    - Straps are secure but not tight.
    - Mask is over nose and mouth.
13. Oxygen catheter
    - Resident's face is free of nasal discharge.
    - Catheter is secured with tape.
14. Oxygen cannula
    - Nasal prongs are in place in nostrils.
    - Elastic band around head is secure but not tight.

(NOTE: Carefully observe resident's mouth when oxygen is being given. Give oral care more frequently.)

5. GUIDELINES FOR REPORTING

Promptly report to the nurse any changes in a resident's condition. *The following changes should be reported immediately.*

1. Change in mental status.
    - Ability to respond.
    - Increasing agitation.
2. Changes in heart and lung status.
    - Difficulty breathing.
    - Weak, irregular, bounding, very rapid or very slow pulse.
    - Changes in blood pressure.
    - Choking.
3. Changes in skin.
    - Flushed and hot.
    - Cyanosis.
    - Cold and clammy.

4. Sudden changes in ability to move body or an extremity.
5. Signs of infection.
   - Elevation in body temperature.
   - Swelling, redness anywhere on body.
   - Complaints of burning/pain when urinating.
   - Coughing.
   - Drainage from pressure sore or other body opening.
6. Sudden changes in hearing and vision.
7. Pain.
8. Evidence of bleeding.
   - From body opening.
   - Bright blood in urine.
   - Vomiting – bright blood or material resembling coffee grounds.
   - Stool – bright blood or black, shiny, tarry looking feces.

6. GUIDELINES FOR RECORDING (Documenting)

1. Do not use the words normal, good, bad, usual, average. These are subjective and do not mean the same thing to everyone.
2. Avoid labeling behavior with descriptions such as uncooperative. Instead, state exactly what happened. For example, "refused to eat lunch."
3. Always use ink in color specified by the facility.

4. Never make erasures or use whiteout on a resident's medical records. Cross through mistaken entry, write "error" above it, and then make correct entry.
5. Use only abbreviations approved by the facility.
6. Do not leave spaces or empty lines between entries.
7. All entries must be dated and have the time when the entry was made.
8. Do not record a procedure or treatment until procedure or treatment has been completed.
9. Do not use the word "resident" when documenting. All the information in the record is about the resident.
10. Include complaints of resident, such as, "complains of sharp pain in left ankle when walking."
11. Sign documentation with your first initial, last name, and status. For example, J. Smith, CNA.

Procedures

TABLE OF CONTENTS

SECTION I: PROCEDURES

1. GUIDELINES FOR PERFORMING NURSING PROCEDURES

As you perform your duties as a nursing assistant, remember to:

1. Perform in a safe manner. Prevent incidents/accidents to residents and to yourself.
2. Perform all principles of medical asepsis, including universal precautions. Prevent the spread of infections among residents, employees, and visitors.
3. Make observations as you work with residents. Report and record accurately and promptly.
4. Work as efficiently as possible. Save steps and energy when you can safely do so without sacrificing quality of care.
5. Be economical of supplies. Use what you need but avoid wastefulness and carelessness. Take care of equipment.
6. Think of the resident as a whole person. Be sensitive to resident's feelings and emotions.

■ BEGINNING PROCEDURE ACTIONS

Before beginning each procedure, complete the following actions:

1. Wash your hands. Wear gloves for procedures involving contact with blood and/or body fluids.
2. Go to the resident's room, knock, and pause before entering.

3. Introduce yourself and identify the resident by checking the resident's identification bracelet.
4. Ask visitors to leave and inform them where they can wait. If resident wishes a family member to stay, allow them to do so, if possible.
5. Provide privacy by closing the door and pulling the cubicle curtain around the bed. Never expose residents unnecessarily.
6. Explain what will happen and answer questions.
7. Raise bed to comfortable working height and lower siderail on side you are working from. Lock wheels of bed.
8. When performing personal care or mobility procedures, permit resident to do as much as he/she is capable of doing.

➡ PROCEDURE COMPLETION ACTIONS

After completing each procedure, complete the following actions:

1. Position resident comfortably.
2. Leave signal cord, telephone, and fresh water close at hand.
3. Return bed to lowest position and raise siderails if necessary.
4. Open cubicle curtains and leave door open unless resident requests that it be closed.
5. Make sure resident has access to any items that might be needed.

6. Clean and store all equipment according to facility policy.
7. Discard all disposable equipment appropriately and promptly.
8. Perform general safety check of resident and environment.
9. Remove gloves and discard. Wash your hands.
10. Ask resident if you can get anything or do anything more before leaving the room.
11. Let visitors know when they may reenter the room.
12. Report completion of task.
13. Document: Name of procedure, time it was completed, reaction of resident, results of procedure, and observations.

ICON

This symbol is used at the beginning and end of each procedure to remind you to perform all beginning procedure actions and all procedure completion actions.

ACTIVITIES OF DAILY LIVING

Activities of daily living include all tasks that adults do every day to meet their basic human needs. These include:

1. Mobility skills
   - Moving in bed
   - Transferring from one surface to another
   - Walking or propelling wheelchair

2. Grooming/hygiene
   ■ Bathing
   ■ Hair care
   ■ Shaving, applying makeup, deodorant
   ■ Nail care
3. Eating
4. Toileting
5. Dressing and undressing

Help residents maintain or regain these skills by remembering the following guidelines:

1. Stress residents' abilities rather than disabilities.
2. Use residents' strengths.
3. Activity strengthens and inactivity weakens. Assist and encourage residents to take part in mental and physical activities.
4. Know what goals have been established for residents.
5. Understand what you need to do to help residents reach these goals.
6. Be sensitive to residents' feelings.
7. Use adaptive equipment appropriately (Figures I-1 and I-2).

Special techniques may help residents regain skills in activities of daily living:

1. Verbal cues
   ■ Set up equipment that resident needs to complete the task.
   ■ Give one word or short phrase to give resident directions. For example:

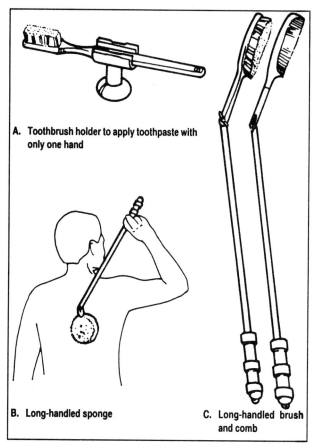

A. Toothbrush holder to apply toothpaste with only one hand

B. Long-handled sponge

C. Long-handled brush and comb

FIGURE I-1. Adaptive devices to aid in personal care *(From Badasch and Chesebro,* Essentials for the Nursing Assistant in Long-Term Care,*1990, Delmar Publishers Inc.)*

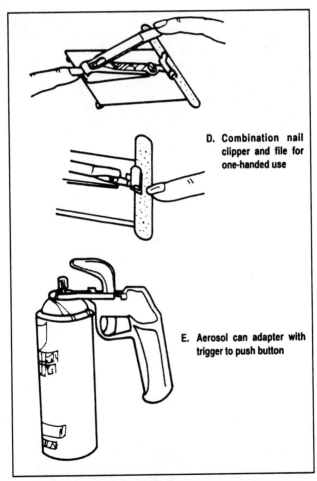

D. Combination nail clipper and file for one-handed use

E. Aerosol can adapter with trigger to push button

FIGURE I-1. Adaptive devices to aid in personal care (continued) *(From Badasch and Chesebro,* Essentials for the Nursing Assistant in Long-Term Care, *1990, Delmar Publishers Inc.)*

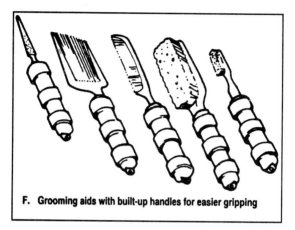

F. Grooming aids with built-up handles for easier gripping

FIGURE I-1. Adaptive devices to aid in personal care (continued) *(From Badasch and Chesebro,* Essentials for the Nursing Assistant in Long-Term Care, *1990, Delmar Publishers Inc.)*

> — "Here is your washcloth" (hand washcloth).
> — "Now wash your face."

2. Hand-over-hand technique
   ■ Place item in resident's hand. For example:
   — Drinking glass, comb, toothbrush.
   ■ Place your hand over resident's hand and guide resident through steps of task.
3. Demonstration
   ■ Use motions to indicate what you want resident to do. For example:
   — Take toothbrush and make motions of brushing your teeth.
   ■ Give toothbrush to resident to imitate your motions.

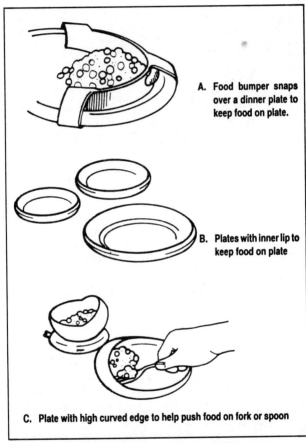

A. Food bumper snaps over a dinner plate to keep food on plate.

B. Plates with inner lip to keep food on plate

C. Plate with high curved edge to help push food on fork or spoon

FIGURE I-2. Adaptive aids to help with eating and drinking *(From Badasch and Chesebro,* Essentials for the Nursing Assistant in Long-Term Care, *1990, Delmar Publishers Inc.)*

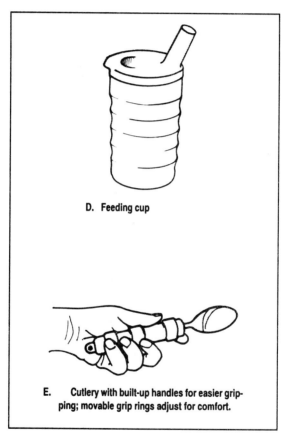

D. Feeding cup

E.   Cutlery with built-up handles for easier grip-
      ping; movable grip rings adjust for comfort.

FIGURE I-2.   Adaptive aids to help with eating and drinking
(continued) *(From Badasch and Chesebro,* Essentials for the
Nursing Assistant in Long-Term Care,*1990, Delmar Publishers
Inc.)*

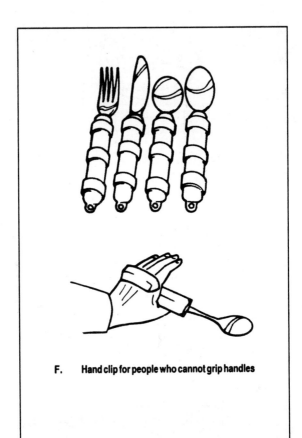

F.   Hand clip for people who cannot grip handles

FIGURE I-2. Adaptive aids to help with eating and drinking (continued) *(From Badasch and Chesebro,* Essentials for the Nursing Assistant in Long-Term Care,*1990, Delmar Publishers Inc.)*

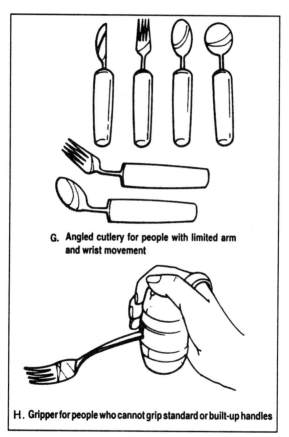

G. Angled cutlery for people with limited arm and wrist movement

H. Gripper for people who cannot grip standard or built-up handles

FIGURE I-2.   Adaptive aids to help with eating and drinking (continued) *(From Badasch and Chesebro,* Essentials for the Nursing Assistant in Long-Term Care, *1990, Delmar Publishers Inc.)*

━━━━━━━━━ **A** ━━━━━━━━━

1. ALTERNATING PRESSURE MATTRESS (Air Mattress)

Purpose of procedure: To reduce pressure against the body so that no skin area is subject to pressure for more than a few minutes at a time.

1. Perform beginning procedure actions.
2. Assemble equipment:
   - Alternating pressure mattress
   - Tubing and pump
   - Two sheets
   - Blanket as needed and bed spread
   - Pillowcases
3. Connect pump to mattress tubing and plug pump in electrical outlet.
4. Place alternating pressure mattress on top of regular mattress. Tuck in only head and foot flaps.
5. Place sheet over both mattresses and tuck in loosely. (Fitted sheets may not fit—a flat sheet can be used.)
6. Never use pins on or near mattress.
7. Check pressure mattress tubing and motor to be sure it is operating properly at least once a shift.
8. Clean pressure mattress with warm water and soap. Rinse well and dry thoroughly.
9. Never disconnect tubing from mattress. Disconnect at motor only.

10. Perform procedure completion actions.

2. AMBULATION

Purpose of procedure: To help resident walk safely.

 1. Perform beginning procedure actions.
2. Assemble equipment:
    - Transfer (gait) belt if needed
    - Resident's shoes and socks if not already on
3. General guidelines:
    - Check if resident is on restorative program to learn mobility skills. Follow directions of program.
    - Always use transfer (gait) belt if resident has problems with balance, coordination, or strength. (See Transfer Belt, Procedure #59.)
    - If resident has balance problems, there should be two people to ambulate resident so counterbalance is provided.
    - If resident's endurance is doubtful, ask another person to follow behind with wheelchair.
    - Resident should always wear sturdy, properly fitting shoes with nonslip soles.
    - Check clothing to be sure shoelaces or slacks are not inhibiting safe ambulation.
    - Place bed in lowest horizontal position.
    - Bring resident to standing position according to care plan instructions.

4. Stand on resident's weaker side.
   ▪ Place your hand closest to resident in back of transfer belt with underhand grasp.
   ▪ Place your far hand on front of resident's shoulder.
5. When resident sits down, be sure chair is touching back of resident's legs.
6. Resident's hands should be placed on arms of chair to lower resident's body into chair.
7. Help resident assume comfortable position in chair.
 8. Perform procedure completion actions.

3. ASSISTING RESIDENT WHO AMBULATES WITH CANE OR WALKER

Purpose of procedure: To help resident walk safely with an assistive device (walker or cane).

 1. Perform beginning procedure actions.
2. Assemble equipment:
   ▪ Transfer (gait) belt if needed
   ▪ Walker or cane
   ▪ Resident's shoes and socks if not already on
3. Check walker or cane for worn areas or loose parts. Be sure rubber tips and hand grips have adequate tread, are not cracked or worn.
4. Follow guidelines from previous procedure for ambulation.
5. Place cane or walker close by.
6. Lower bed to lowest horizontal position. Assist resident to stand. Resident should not use walker to bring self to standing position.

7. Hand resident cane or place walker in front within resident's reach.
8. The cane is held on the strong side. Resident should advance cane 10–18 inches followed by weaker leg and then strong leg.
9. For using a walker, have resident advance walker about 10–18 inches. Resident then should move weaker leg forward into walker followed by stronger leg. All four points of walker should strike floor at same time.
10. If resident has transfer belt on, stand on resident's weaker side and slightly in back with your hands in the belt.
11. After ambulation, return resident to bed or chair.
    ■ Have resident walk within a step of bed or chair.
    ■ Place cane or walker to side and assist resident to turn around.
    ■ When resident feels bed or chair touching back of legs, have resident reach for the arm of chair or mattress of bed and lower self into chair or bed.

 12. Perform procedure completion actions.

4. AQUAMATIC K-PAD®

Purpose of procedure: To apply dry heat with constant temperature to a specific body part.

 1. Perform beginning procedure actions.
2. Assemble equipment:
    ■ Aquamatic K-Pad®and control unit

■ Distilled water
■ Covering for pad
3. Place control unit on bedside stand.
4. Remove cover and fill unit with distilled water to fill line.
5. Screw cover in place and loosen one-quarter turn.
6. Note time of application. Turn on unit. If temperature has not been preset, set to 95–100°F. Remove key after setting.
7. Cover pad and place on resident.
   ■ Secure with tape.
   ■ Never use pins.
   ■ Be sure tubing is coiled on bed to facilitate flow.
   ■ Do not allow tubing to hang below level of bed.
8. Periodically check control unit. Refill unit if water drops below fill line.
9. Remove pad after prescribed period of time.
 10. Perform procedure completion actions.

5. ARTIFICIAL EYE CARE

Purpose of procedure: To maintain cleanliness of artificial eye.

1. Perform beginning procedure actions.
2. Assemble equipment:
   ■ Eyecup lined with gauze
   ■ Cotton balls
   ■ Washcloth
   ■ Lukewarm water
   ■ Cleansing solution if ordered

3. Assist resident into bed.
4. Have resident close eyes and turn head to side of prosthesis.
5. Wash outside eye with warm water, using one cotton ball at a time. Stroke only once with each cotton ball from inner eye to outer eye.
6. Remove eye by depressing lower eyelid with your thumb while lifting upper lid with your finger.
   - Take eye in your hand.
   - Place in eyecup.
   - Place eyecup and prosthesis in center of bedside stand.
7. Clean eye socket using warm water and cotton balls. Dry area around eye gently.
8. Carry eyecup to bathroom.
   - Clean sink.
   - Fill sink half full with lukewarm water.
   - Place folded washcloth in bottom of sink.
   - Remove eye from eyecup and place in water in sink.
   - Use no abrasives or general solvents.
9. Empty water from eyecup.
   - Place fresh gauze square on bottom of eyecup.
   - Place wet eye on gauze.
   - Add water if eye is to be stored in drawer of bedside stand.
10. Wash your hands and return to bedside to reinsert eye.
11. Depress lower lid and slip over prosthesis.
12. Perform procedure completion actions.

■ B ■

6. BATH, CENTURY TUB

Purpose of procedure: To provide all the benefits of bathing as well as the additional benefit of whirlpool activity.

1. Perform beginning procedure actions.
2. Assemble equipment:
   - Two bath towels
   - One bath blanket
   - Deodorant (optional)
   - Talcum powder (optional)
   - Resident's clothing
3. Prepare bath before transporting resident to bath area.
   - Be sure tub is clean and fill with water at 97°F to approximately 8 inches from top.
   - Room temperature should be about 70° F.
   - Add one capful of liquid soap or as facility policy states.
4. Get Saf-Kary®chair and take to bedside.
5. Help resident undress.
6. Position resident in Saf-Kary®chair. Secure safety straps and cover resident with bath blanket.
7. Transport resident to tub room.
8. Replace bath blanket with two towels. Fold blanket for later use.
9. Position chair with back against lift arms.

10. Step on *up* pedal of lift to engage seat on Saf-Kary®chair.
11. Check that both pins are engaged in lift arm slots.
12. Latch safety latches.
13. Raise seat to maximum height.
14. Rotate seat on lift arm 90 degrees so resident faces you.
15. Facing resident, slowly guide chair to tub edge so resident is parallel and over tub edge.
16. Lift resident's feet and guide them over tub edge toward lower well of tub.
17. Lower resident into tub by stepping gently on *down* pedal. Water should be chest high.
18. Press turbine button, activating whirlpool for five minutes.
19. Bathe face and upper body.
20. Step on *up* pedal, raising resident until feet are level with whirlpool outlet.
21. Dry upper body.
22. Raise lift to maximum height.
23. Pull chair and resident toward you, rotating seat as you lift feet from tub. Dry feet and legs.
24. Cover resident with bath towel.
25. Raise safety latch on Saf-Kary®chair.
26. Apply deodorant and talcum powder if resident desires.
27. Help resident dress.
28. Slowly lower lift and Saf-Kary®chair until it is flat on floor.
29. Return resident to unit.
30. Return to tub room and clean tub according to facility policy.

31. Perform procedure completion actions.

7. BATH, EMOLLIENT

Purpose of procedure: To soothe and treat a skin condition. A substance such as baking soda, cornstarch, or oatmeal is added.

 1. Perform beginning procedure actions.
2. Assemble equipment:
    - Bath mat
    - Two bath towels and wash cloth
    - Disposable gloves
    - Gown
    - Robe and slippers
    - Bath thermometer
    - Additions as ordered
3. Be sure tub is clean and room is comfortably warm.
4. Fill tub with water at 95–100°F. Check temperature with bath thermometer.
5. Add medication if ordered and stir well.
6. Transfer resident to tub as outlined in tub bath procedure.
7. Have resident lie in tub for 30 minutes to one hour as ordered.
    - Gently sponge areas not covered with water.
    - Make sure resident does not become chilled.
    - Add warm water as needed.
8. Assist resident out of tub. Dry skin by patting with soft towel. *Do not rub.*

9. Apply lotion if ordered by patting.
10. Assist resident to bed and encourage resident to rest.
11. Clean tub and replace equipment according to facility policy.
 12. Perform procedure completion actions.

8. BLADDER AND BOWEL RETRAINING PROCEDURES

Purpose of procedure: To assist resident to restore bladder and/or bowel function, eliminating incontinence.

(**NOTE:** This procedure takes from 6–8 weeks and requires the cooperation of all staff and resident. It is initiated only after careful evaluation by the registered nurse.)

 1. Perform procedure actions.
2. Assemble equipment:
   - Incontinence record
   - Intake and output record
   - Other items as required for specific resident
3. Enlist resident's cooperation.
4. Make a record of resident's incontinence times.
5. Provide resident with opportunity to void according to schedule established by nurse.
   - During night, keep urinal at bedside for males, take resident to bathroom, or offer bedpan.

6. Fluid control may be initiated after 7:00 PM. Follow facility policy.
7. Assist resident to appropriate position during voiding.
    - Resident should be sitting upright with hips and knees flexed, and feet flat on floor.
    - A height of 20 inches is most satisfactory for toilet seat. A device for raising height and providing handrails may be applied to toilet.
    - Men find it easier to void in standing position. They may require support.
    - If resident uses bedpan, position resident comfortably.
    - A fracture pan may be more comfortable.
8. Additional stimuli may start flow of urine and help empty bladder:
    - Offer glass of water to drink.
    - Pour measured warm water over perineum.
    - Help resident lean forward. Gently stroke inner thigh.
    - Run water in sink so resident can hear it.
    - Place resident's hand in warm water.
    - Encourage resident to bear down at end of voiding to completely empty bladder. *This may be contraindicated for some residents, especially those with heart problems.*
9. Measure and record output.
10. Perform procedure completion actions.

9. BLOOD PRESSURE

Purpose of procedure: To keep record of resident's blood pressure.

 1. Perform beginning procedure actions.
   2. Assemble equipment:
      ▪ Sphygmomanometer (blood pressure cuff with gauge)

(NOTE: Be sure to use correct size of cuff for residents with very large or very small arms. Using the wrong size results in an incorrect reading.)

      ▪ Stethoscope
      ▪ Alcohol pads
      ▪ Pad and pencil
   3. Place resident's arm with palm up, supported on bed, arm of chair or table.
   4. Roll sleeve up about five inches above elbow. Be sure it is not tight.
   5. Apply cuff smoothly and evenly 1 to 1-1/2 inches above elbow. Center of rubber bladder should be directly over brachial artery. If cuff is marked with arrow, place cuff so arrow points over brachial artery.
   6. Tuck ends of cuff under a fold or hook or use Velcro closure. Be sure cuff is secure but not too tight.
   7. Locate radial artery and palpate it as you:
      ▪ Close valve attached to air bulb by turning clockwise.
      ▪ Quickly inflate cuff until gauge registers 50 mm Hg.
      ▪ Continue to inflate cuff in 10 mm Hg increments until radial pulse cannot be felt. Note pressure.

8. Quickly deflate cuff by turning valve counterclockwise.
9. Ask resident to raise arm and flex fingers.
10. Locate brachial artery with fingers.
11. Place earpieces of stethoscope in ears. Place bell of stethoscope directly over artery.
12. Close valve and reinflate cuff quickly until gauge registers 30 mm Hg above palpated systolic pressure.
13. Carefully listen as you open valve of bulb by turning counterclockwise.
14. Let air escape slowly until first heart sound is heard. Note reading on gauge as systolic pressure.
15. Continue to slowly release air pressure until there is an abrupt change of sound from very loud to soft muffled sound. The reading at which this change is heard is diastolic pressure. In some facilities, the last sound heard is taken as diastolic pressure.
16. Rapidly deflate cuff and remove, expel air from cuff and replace apparatus. Clean earpieces and bell of stethoscope with alcohol pads.

(NOTE: If procedure must be repeated, wait at least one minute. Ask resident to raise arm and flex fingers. Repeat procedure.)

▶ 17. Perform procedure completion actions.

(NOTE: Report to nurse if unable to hear reading or if reading is significantly higher or lower than last reading.)

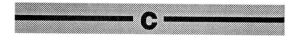

10. CAST CARE

Purpose of procedure: To promote adequate circulation and to observe for decreased circulation in the casted extremity.

   1. Perform beginning procedure actions.
   2. Assemble equipment:
      - Pillows
      - Pillow cases
      - Plastic pillow covers
   3. Care of newly casted resident:
      - Support cast and body in good alignment with pillows covered with plastic cover and cloth pillow case. Keep cast uncovered.
      - Observe toes or fingers of casted extremity for coldness, cyanosis, swelling, or numbness. If present, immediately notify nurse.
      - Use palms of hands not fingers if cast must be moved.
      - Check skin areas around cast edges for signs of irritation. Notify nurse if edges of cast need to be taped or padded.
   4. Care after cast is dry:
      - Turn resident according to care-plan instructions.
      - Always support cast.
      - Encourage use of overhead bar (trapeze) to assist resident in helping self.

- Check toes or fingers of casted extremity for circulation as directed above.
- Check skin areas around edges of cast as directed above.
- Use plastic during elimination to protect cast edges that are near genitals and buttocks to prevent soiling from urine or feces.
- Check with nurse for bathing procedures. You may be able to wrap casted extremity in plastic bag so resident can have a shower.

 5. Perform procedure completion actions.

11. CATHETER CARE

Purpose of procedure: To prevent urinary tract infections.

 1. Perform beginning procedure actions.
2. Assemble equipment:
   - Disposable gloves
   - Bed protector
   - Bath blanket
   - Plastic bag for disposables
   - Daily catheter care kit
   - Antiseptic solution
   - Sterile applicators
   - Catheter strap

(**NOTE:** Many facilities only do routine care for residents with catheters, the same as would be done for residents without catheters. The need for antiseptic application is questionable. Follow facility policy.)

3. Be sure opposite siderail is up and secure. Cover resident with bath blanket and fanfold bedding to foot of bed.
4. Position resident on back, legs separated, and knees bent, if possible.
5. Position bath blanket so only genitals are exposed.
6. Ask resident to raise hips and place bed protector under resident.
7. Arrange catheter care kit and plastic bag on over-bed table. Open kit.
8. Put on gloves and draw drape back.
9. For male resident:
   - Gently grasp penis and draw foreskin back.
   - Using applicator dipped in antiseptic solution, cleanse glans from meatus toward shaft for about four inches. Use applicator for only one stroke.
   - Dispose of each used applicator in plastic bag after one stroke.
10. For female resident:
    - Separate labia.
    - Using applicator dipped in antiseptic, stroke from front to back. Use applicator for only one stroke. Dispose of each used applicator in plastic bag after one stroke.
11. Remove gloves and discard in plastic bag.
12. Check catheter to be sure it is secured with catheter strap. Replace strap if necessary. (Tape may be used but may be harmful to an elderly person's fragile skin.)

13. Check to be sure tubing is coiled on bed and hangs straight down into drainage container. End of tubing should not be below level of urine in container. Empty bag and measure if necessary. Do not raise bag above level of bladder (Figure I-3).

14. Replace bedding and remove bath blanket. Fold and leave in bedside stand.

 15. Perform procedure completion actions.

12. CATHETER, DISCONNECTING

Purpose of procedure: To prevent contamination of catheter setup when drainage system must be disconnected.

(**NOTE:** It is preferable to never disconnect drainage setup, but sometimes this may be necessary. If sterile caps and plugs are available they should be used. If not, the disconnected ends must be protected with sterile gauze sponges.

 1. Perform beginning procedure actions.

2. Assemble equipment:
   - Alcohol pads
   - Disposable gloves
   - Gauze sponges
   - Sterile caps/plugs
   - Clamps
   - Plastic bag

3. Clamp catheter just above Y site.

4. Disinfect area to be disconnected with alcohol pad. Put on gloves.

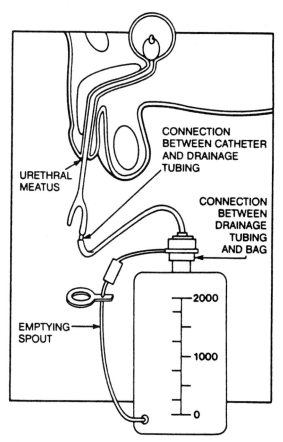

FIGURE I-3. Protect possible sites of contamination in closed urinary drainage system by keeping drainage bag below level of bladder. *(From Caldwell and Hegner,* Nursing Assistant, A Nursing Process Approach, *5th Edition, 1989, Delmar Publishers Inc.)*

5. Disconnect catheter and drainage tubing. Do not put them down or allow them to touch anything.
6. Insert sterile plug in end of catheter (Figure I-4). Place sterile cap over exposed end of drainage tube.
7. Secure drainage tube to bed so it will not touch floor.
8. Remove gloves and dispose of in plastic bag.
 9. Perform procedure completion actions.

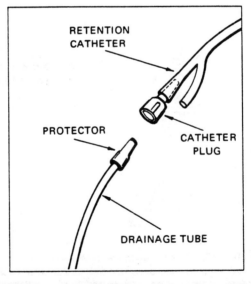

FIGURE I-4. Plug and protective cap in place *(From Caldwell and Hegner,* Nursing Assistant, A Nursing Process Approach, *5th Edition, 1989, Delmar Publishers Inc.)*

13. CATHETER, EMPTYING DRAINAGE UNIT

Purpose of procedure: To prevent odors from urine in drainage container and to maintain accurate records of residents' urinary output.

 1. Perform beginning procedure actions.
  2. Assemble equipment:
     - Graduate container
     - Disposable gloves
     - Sterile cap or sterile gauze sponge (needed if container has no bottom drain tube)
     - Plastic bag
     - Alcohol pad
  3. Put on gloves.
  4. If drainage bag has drain in bottom, place graduate under it.
  5. Open drain and allow urine to drain into graduate. Do not allow tip of tubing to touch sides of graduate.
  6. Close drain and wipe with alcohol pad. Replace it in holder.
  7. If there is no opening, tube must be removed before emptying. Protect end of drainage tube with sterile cap or sterile sponge.
  8. Empty urine into graduate.
  9. Remove protective cover from end of tube. Reinsert tube into bag. Be careful not to touch sides of bag with tip of tube.
 10. Note amount and character of urine.
 11. Check position of drainage tube.
 12. Take graduate (covered) to utility room and empty.
 13. Remove gloves and dispose of in plastic bag.

14. Perform procedure completion actions.

14. CATHETER WITH LEG BAG

Purpose of procedure: To allow residents with indwelling catheters more freedom of movement. These directions are for connecting regular drainage tube and collection bag and then attaching leg bag to catheter.

(**NOTE:** Leg bag is worn only when resident is ambulatory or sitting in chair. Leg bag is removed and regular drainage tubing and bag are reconnected when resident is in bed.)

 1. Perform beginning procedure actions.
   2. Assemble equipment:
      - Disposable gloves
      - Alcohol pads
      - Sterile caps
      - Catheter clamp
   3. Attach leg bag to resident's leg.
      - A small folded towel may be placed around leg and under straps of leg bag to avoid skin irritation.
      - Make sure drainage opening is at bottom and that cap is secure.
      - Adjust straps so they are secure but not too tight.
   4. Put on gloves.
   5. Swab attachment site of catheter and drainage tube with alcohol pad. Clamp catheter.

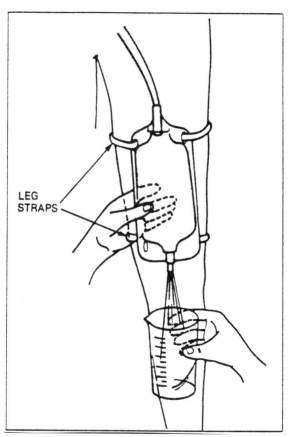

FIGURE I-5. Catheter is connected to top opening of leg bag. Leg bag is drained from bottom opening. *(From Badasch and Chesebro, Essentials for the Nursing Assistant in Long-Term Care, 1990, Delmar Publishers Inc.)*

6. Disconnect catheter and drainage tubing. Do not put them down or allow them to touch anything.
7. Place sterile cap over end of drainage tubing.
8. Position end of drainage tubing so it will not touch floor.
9. Remove cap from opening of leg bag and connect catheter to this opening (Figure I-5).
10. Remove catheter clamp.
11. Empty regular drainage bag and care for tubing and drainage bag according to facility policy.
12. Remove and dispose of gloves.
13. Check leg bag frequently and empty when necessary. To empty:
    ■ Put on disposable gloves.
    ■ Swab drainage opening of leg bag with alcohol pad.
    ■ Drain urine into graduate container. Check whether specimen is needed.
    ■ Recap drainage opening of bag.
    ■ Dispose of urine after measuring.
    ■ Remove and dispose of gloves. Wash hands.
14. Perform procedure completion actions.

15. COLD PACK (Disposable)

Purpose of procedure: To apply dry cold to an area of the body to reduce swelling; to numb sensation of pain; to reduce inflammation or itching.

1. Perform beginning procedure actions.
2. Assemble equipment:
    - Disposable cold pack (commercially prepared). Read directions.
    - Clean covering (towel or hot water bag cover)
    - Tape or rolls of gauze
3. Expose body area to be treated. Note condition of area.
4. Place cold pack in cloth cover.
5. Strike or squeeze cold pack to activate chemicals.
6. Place covered cold pack on proper area and enclose with towel. Note time of application.
7. Secure with tape or gauze.
8. Leave resident in comfortable position with signal cord within easy reach.
9. Return to resident every 10 minutes. Check area being treated for discoloration or numbness. If these occur, discontinue treatment and report them to nurse.
10. If no adverse symptoms occur, remove pack in 30 minutes. Note condition of area. Continuous treatment requires application of fresh pack.
11. Remove pack from cover and discard according to facility policy. Return unused gauze and tape. Put cover in laundry.
12. Perform procedure completion actions.

16. COLOSTOMY, ROUTINE STOMA CARE

Purpose of procedure: To clean stomal area of feces and drainage so odors and skin breakdown are prevented (Figure I-6).

1. Perform beginning procedure actions.
2. Assemble equipment:
   - Washcloth and towel
   - Basin of warm water
   - Bed protector
   - Bath blanket
   - Disposable colostomy bag and belt
   - Bedpan
   - Disposable gloves
   - Skin lotion as directed
3. Replace top bedding with bath blanket.
4. Place bed protector under resident's hips.
5. Put on disposable gloves.
6. Remove soiled disposable stoma bag and place in bedpan. Note amount and type of drainage.
7. Remove belt that holds stoma bag and save if clean.
8. Gently clean area around stoma with toilet tissue to remove feces and drainage. Dispose of tissue in bedpan.
9. Wash area around stoma with soap and water. Rinse thoroughly and dry.
10. If ordered, apply skin lotion lightly around stoma. (Too much lotion may interfere with proper adhesion of fresh ostomy bag.)
11. Position clean belt around resident. Inspect area for irritation or breakdown.

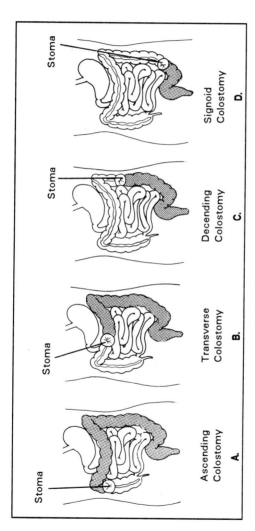

FIGURE I-6. Colostomy sites *(From Caldwell and Hegner, Nursing Assistant, A Nursing Process Approach, 5th Edition, 1989, Delmar Publishers Inc.)*

12. If necessary, remove and replace adhesive wafer. Place clean ostomy bag over stoma and secure belt.

13. Remove bed protector. Check to be sure bottom bedding is not wet. Change if necessary.

14. Replace bath blanket with top bedding, making resident comfortable.

15. Perform procedure completion actions.

16. Gather soiled materials and bedpan. Take to utility room and dispose of according to facility policy. Empty, wash, and dry bedpan. Return it to resident's unit.

17. COOLING BATH

Purpose of procedure: To reduce a resident's temperature when it is very elevated and unresponsive to other treatments.

(NOTE: This procedure is too drastic for children and elderly people. The procedure should be closely supervised by the nurse.)

1. Perform beginning procedure actions.

2. Assemble equipment:
   - Two bath towels
   - One hand towel
   - Two bath blankets
   - Two washcloths
   - One hot water bag
   - Six cloth-covered ice bags or disposable ice packs
   - Thermometer (for body temperature)
   - Bath thermometer
   - Basin
   - Clean gown

■ Bed protector
3. Lower siderail on your side.
4. Take resident's temperature, pulse, and respirations. Note time and readings.
5. Cover resident with bath blanket. Remove gown. Fanfold top bedding to foot of bed.
6. Position bath blanket under resident.
7. Put up siderails.
8. Prepare hot water bag and ice packs. Place in cloth covers.
9. Fill basin with water and alcohol, if ordered:
    ■ Dilution of alcohol to water should be 1:1 unless otherwise ordered.
    ■ Add ice cubes if ordered.
    ■ Check temperature with bath thermometer.
10. Return to bedside with equipment. Lower siderail nearest you and position resident close to you.
11. Fold small towel lengthwise and position over genitalia.
12. Place covered hot water bag at resident's feet.
13. Place covered ice bags:
    ■ On the head.
    ■ In each axilla.
    ■ On the groin.
    ■ On either side of neck if ordered.
14. Place washcloths in solution.
    ■ Alternate washcloths.
    ■ Wring out tightly so solution will not drip.
15. Expose far arm.
    ■ Place bath towel or bed protector lengthwise underneath it.

■ Sponge arm for five minutes.
■ Do not dry.
■ Cover with bath blanket upon completion.

16. Repeat procedure with near arm.
17. Place bath towel over resident's chest and abdomen. Fold bath blanket to abdomen.
18. Bathe neck, shoulders, and chest for five minutes.
19. Fold bath blanket to groin and bathe abdomen.
20. Expose far leg and place towel lengthwise under it.
    ■ Bathe leg for five minutes.
    ■ Cover with bath blanket.
    ■ Remove towel.
21. Repeat procedure with leg nearest you.
22. Assist resident to turn away from you.
23. Place towel on bed along back. Bathe back for five minutes.
24. Position resident on back.
25. Remove hot water bag, ice packs, and bath blanket from under resident.
26. Change bottom linen if necessary.
27. Replace gown and top bedding. Remove bath blanket.
28. Take temperature, pulse, and respirations. Make notation of time and readings.
29. Perform procedure completion actions.
30. Return to bedside 30 minutes later to measure temperature, pulse, and respirations.
31. Report results to nurse.
32. Perform procedure completion actions.

━━━━━■ **D** ■━━━━━

18. DRESSING AND UNDRESSING RESIDENT

Purpose of procedure: To dress resident so he/she is comfortable and attractive; to avoid incidents due to unsafe unclothing. To undress resident in preparation for bathing or bedtime.

GENERAL GUIDELINES FOR DRESSING AND UNDRESSING

1. All residents who are out of bed should be dressed.
2. Assess resident's mental and physical condition and ability to assist in procedure.
3. Allow resident choices of clothing if possible.
4. Be sure that clothing is in good repair, clean, and matched. It should be appropriate for climate and resident's sex, age, and personality.
5. Demonstrate respect for all clothing. Do not cut, tear, or damage. Store clothing neatly.
6. Residents should wear underwear when they are dressed, unless care plan indicates otherwise.
7. Residents who will be transferring or ambulating should have socks and well-fitting shoes with nonslip soles.
8. Check if resident is on restorative program to relearn dressing/undressing skills. If so, follow directions for program. Use adaptive devices correctly (Figure I-7).

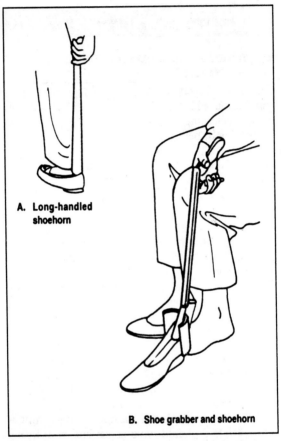

A. Long-handled shoehorn

B. Shoe grabber and shoehorn

FIGURE I-7. Dressing aids *(From Badasch and Chesebro, Essentials for the Nursing Assistant in Long-Term Care, 1990, Delmar Publishers Inc.)*

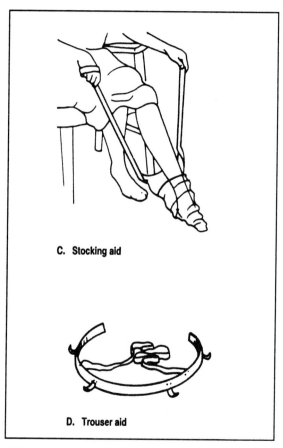

C. Stocking aid

D. Trouser aid

FIGURE I-7. Dressing aids (continued) *(From Badasch and Chesebro,* Essentials for the Nursing Assistant in Long-Term Care, *1990, Delmar Publishers Inc.)*

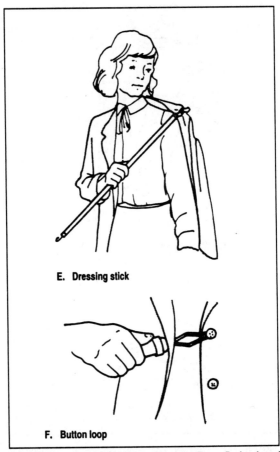

E. Dressing stick

F. Button loop

FIGURE I-7. Dressing aids (continued) *(From Badasch and Chesebro, Essentials for the Nursing Assistant in Long-Term Care, 1990, Delmar Publishers Inc.)*

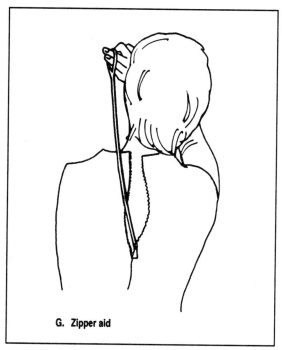

G. Zipper aid

FIGURE I-7. Dressing aids (continued) *(From Badasch and Chesebro,* Essentials for the Nursing Assistant in Long-Term Care, *1990, Delmar Publishers Inc.)*

9. All clothing brought into the facility for residents on admission or later should be labeled with resident's name. Label should be concealed in inner part of garment.

(NOTE: Instructions are given for various types of garments.)

Before dressing and undressing residents:

➡ 10. Perform beginning procedure actions.
   11. Assemble clothing that is needed and lay it
       out for easy access.

CHANGING A GOWN

1. Loosen gown from neck.
2. Slip gown down over arms. Remove from
   arms without exposing resident. Place clean
   gown over resident's chest and hold it in
   place while you slide soiled gown out from
   underneath.
3. Slide sleeves up over resident's arms. Fasten gown.

NOTE: If IV line is in place:

4. Remove gown from arm without IV first.
5. Slip gown down over arm with IV.
6. Gather gown at arm and slip downward over
   arm and line.
7. Gather material of gown in one hand and
   slowly draw gown over tips of fingers.
8. With free hand, lift IV free of standard and
   slip gown over bottle. Do not lower bottle at
   any time. Raise gown up over bottle and
   replace bottle on standard.

To put on gown with IV line in place:

9. Gather sleeve on IV side in one hand.
10. Lift bottle free of standard, maintaining
    height.
11. Slip IV bottle through sleeve from inside
    and rehang.

12. Guide gown along IV tubing to bed.
13. Slip gown carefully over hand.
14. Position gown on infusion arm. Then insert opposite arm.

PULLOVER GARMENTS

Undressing:

1. Unbutton or spread neck opening.
2. If garment is big enough or made of stretchy fabric:
   - Gather garment in back with your hand and ease up to neck and up over back of resident's head.
   - Slide garment down over resident's head and face.
   - Using both hands, gently pull garment down over both resident's arms and hands, removing garment completely.
3. If previous method is not possible:
   - Remove stronger arm from garment first.
   - Grasp sleeve at lower edge, support arm, remove sleeve.
   - Repeat to remove sleeve from weaker arm.
   - Gather front of garment from hem to neckline, slip smoothly over head.
   - Support head and neck with one hand, reach under neck with other hand, grasp garment and pull toward you.
   - Remove garment.

Dressing:
1. Unbutton or spread neck opening.
2. If garment is big enough or made of stretchy fabric:
   ■ Place garment over resident's hands and then pull up over arms as far as possible.
   ■ Spread neck opening and slip over resident's head.
   ■ Pull garment down over resident's trunk, smooth out and adjust.
3. If this method is not possible:
   ■ Spread neck opening and bring down over resident's head.
   ■ Place one of your hands through end of sleeve.
   ■ Support resident's weaker arm with your other hand and ease through sleeve.
   ■ Repeat with other arm.
   ■ Smooth out and adjust garment.

CARDIGAN STYLE GARMENTS

Undressing:
1. Open garment as far as possible.
2. Bring garment down over shoulder of strongest arm and remove arm from sleeve.
3. Bring garment around back of resident (or front if garment is open in back).
4. Support resident's arm and slide down over weaker arm and remove.

Dressing:
1. Open garment as far as possible.
2. Place your hand through sleeve opening and support resident's weaker arm.

3. Slide sleeve up over arm and shoulder.
4. Bring rest of garment around back of resident (or front if garment is open in back).
5. Place resident's strong arm in sleeve, bring
   garment up to shoulder.
6. Smooth out and adjust garment. Fasten.

PANTS/SLACKS

(NOTE: Pants, slacks, and skirts are easier to put on
         with the resident lying in bed, unless the
         resident has good sitting or standing
         balance.)

Undressing:
1. Unfasten clothing. Place towel over lower
   abdomen and thighs.
2. If resident is able to lift buttocks, slip pants
   down to thighs.
3. If resident cannot do this, roll resident on
   side toward you, easing clothing down.
4. Turn resident away from you and ease clothing down on other side.
5. Return resident to back and place one hand
   over each of resident's hips. Gently work
   clothing down over legs toward ankles.
6. Support foot with your hand and ease clothing over foot. Repeat with other foot.

Dressing:
1. Gather most of pant leg in one hand. Clasp
   resident's ankle with other hand and guide
   foot through pant leg.
2. Repeat with other side.
3. Ease pants up over legs, knees, and thighs. If
   resident can raise buttocks, have him do so

while you grasp pants on each side and pull
up to waist.

4. If unable to raise buttocks, reverse procedure for taking pants off.

(NOTE: Skirts may be put on or taken off like
slacks, or over the head like a dress. For
dresses, follow the directions for either
pullover or cardigan style clothing, depending on style of the dress.)

SHOES AND SOCKS

1. To put on socks, gather sock from top to
toes.
2. Slip on over resident's toes and up over heel.
3. Smooth sock up over ankle.
4. To remove socks, reverse procedure.
5. To put on shoes, spread opening as far as
possible if there are laces or Velcro closings.
6. Put shoes on over toes and heel. This is
much easier with a shoehorn.
7. Push shoe from bottom to finish putting it
on. Remove shoehorn.
8. Make sure shoes are on all the way. Fasten
securely.
9. At end of all dressing/undressing procedures,
perform procedure completion actions.

(NOTE: Report to the appropriate person when
resident is in need of new clothing. Follow
facility policy for sending garments to
laundry and for getting garments repaired.)

19. ENEMA, COMMERCIALLY PREPARED

Purpose of procedure: To remove feces and flatus from colon and rectum of resident who is unable to retain large amounts of fluid.

1. Perform beginning procedure actions.
2. Assemble equipment:
   - Disposable prepackaged enema
   - Bedpan and cover or bedside commode
   - Bed protector
   - Toilet tissue
   - Disposable gloves
   - Pan of warm water if enema solution is to be warmed
   - Towel, soap, and basin with warm water
3. Open package and remove plastic container with enema solution. Place solution container in warm water if it is to be warmed.
4. Place bedpan and cover on chair close at hand or position commode next to bed.
5. Lower head of bed. If resident will be using commode, lower bed to lowest horizontal position. Have resident's slippers and robe available or put them on resident before beginning procedure.
6. Assist resident to assume left Sims' position.
7. Place bed protector under resident.
8. Put on disposable gloves.

9. Expose only resident's buttocks by drawing bedding upward in one hand.
10. Remove cover from enema tip.
11. Separate buttocks, exposing anus, and ask resident to breathe in.
12. Insert lubricated enema tip two inches into rectum.
13. Squeeze plastic container slowly from bottom of container until all fluid has entered resident's body.
14. Remove tip from resident and place container in box. Encourage resident to hold solution as long as possible.
15. When resident feels urge to defecate (usually in 5–15 minutes), assist resident to bathroom/commode or position on bedpan.
16. Remove and dispose of gloves.
17. If resident uses bedpan, raise head of bed to comfortable position.
18. Place toilet tissue and signal cord within reach of resident. Raise siderails if resident is on bedpan. If resident is in bathroom or on commode, stay close by. Caution resident not to flush toilet.
19. Return to resident when signaled. Put on gloves. Assist resident to clean perineal and rectal area if necessary.
20. Remove bedpan or assist resident to return to bed.
21. Observe results of enema. Flush stool or cover bedpan or commode. Empty contents of commode or bedpan according to facility policy.

22. Dispose of equipment according to facility policy.
23. Remove gloves and wash hands.
24. Give resident opportunity to wash hands and return equipment.

 25. Perform procedure completion actions.

20. ENEMA, OIL RETENTION

Purpose of procedure: To instill oil into resident's rectum to soften feces. This procedure is usually followed with administration of a soapsuds enema.

 1. Perform beginning procedure actions.
2. Assemble equipment:
   - Bedpan and cover or commode
   - Toilet tissue
   - Towel, soap, basin with water
   - Prepackaged oil enema
   - Bed protector
   - Disposable gloves
3. Instruct resident that it will be necessary to hold solution for at least 20 minutes.
4. Place bedpan with cover on chair close to bed, or place commode close to bed.
5. If resident will be getting up to use bathroom or commode, get slippers and robe or have resident put them on before giving the enema.
6. Lower head of bed if necessary and help resident assume left Sims' position. Place bed protector under buttocks.

7. Open prepackaged oil-retention enema.
8. Put on gloves.
9. Expose only resident's buttocks by drawing bedding upward in one hand.
10. Remove cover from enema tip (Figure I-8).
11. Separate buttocks, exposing anus, and insert prelubricated tip into anus as resident takes deep breath.
12. Squeeze container until all solution has been given.
13. Remove container and place in package box to be discarded.
14. Encourage resident to remain on left side.
15. Remove and dispose of gloves. Wash hands.
16. Check resident every five minutes until fluid has been retained for 20 minutes.
17. Position resident on bedpan or assist to bathroom or commode.
18. Place toilet tissue and signal cord within easy reach of resident. If resident is on commode or in bathroom, stay nearby. Caution resident not to flush toilet.
19. Put on disposable gloves.
20. Remove bedpan or assist resident to return to bed.
    ■ Assist resident to clean perineal and rectal area if necessary.
    ■ Observe results of enema.
    ■ Cover bedpan or commode and dispose of contents or flush toilet.
21. Assist resident to wash and dry hands.
22. Remove bed protector. Clean or dispose of all equipment according to facility policy.
23. Remove and discard gloves. Wash hands.

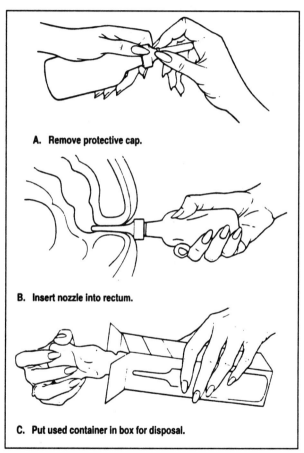

A. Remove protective cap.

B. Insert nozzle into rectum.

C. Put used container in box for disposal.

FIGURE I-8. Administering an oil retention enema *(Courtesy of C.B. Fleet Co., Inc., From Caldwell and Hegner,* Nursing Assistant, A Nursing Process Approach, *5th Edition, 1989, Delmar Publishers Inc.)*

24. Perform procedure completion actions.

21. ENEMA, RETURN FLOW (Harris Flush)

Purpose of procedure: To relieve abdominal distention caused by flatus.

 1. Perform beginning procedure actions.
  2. Assemble equipment:
     - Irrigating can
     - Enema tubing and clamp
     - Lubricant
     - Bed protector
     - Toilet tissue
     - Solution: 500 ml tap water at 105°F
     - Disposable gloves
  3. Put solution into irrigating can.
     - Allow small amount of fluid to run through tubing to remove air.
     - Lubricate end of tubing and place end of tubing on paper towel.
  4. Assist resident to assume left Sims' position and place bed protector under resident's buttocks.
  5. Put on gloves.
  6. Expose only resident's buttocks by drawing bedding upward in one hand.
  7. Separate buttocks, exposing anus, and ask resident to take deep breath.
  8. Insert tube into rectum about four inches.
  9. Handle Harris flush in following way to bring about peristalsis.

- ■ Open clamp, raise irrigating can to height of 12–18 inches above resident's hips and allow about 200 ml of fluid to run into rectum.
- ■ Lower irrigating can about 12 inches above level of bed and allow fluid to flow out of rectum into can.

10. Continue procedure until some gas is expelled. When all fluid has been returned, clamp tube and remove.
11. Use toilet tissue to remove lubricant and moisture from rectal area.
12. Remove bed protector.
13. Remove gloves.
14. Clean or dispose of all equipment according to facility policy.
 15. Perform procedure completion actions.

22. ENEMA, ROTATING

Purpose of procedure: To remove feces and flatus from colon and rectum.

(NOTE: This procedure varies only slightly from regular soapsuds enema. The same equipment is used and about 1000 ml of fluid is allowed to flow into rectum.)

1. Perform beginning procedure actions.
2. Follow Steps 1–8 for soapsuds enema.
3. Raise foot of bed about 30 degrees.
4. Expose only resident's buttocks by drawing bedding upward in one hand.

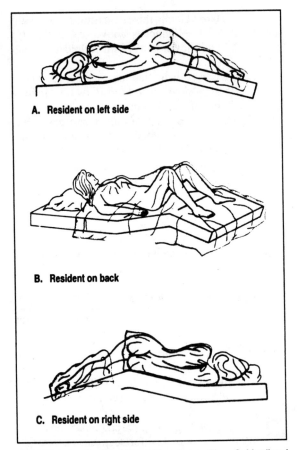

A. Resident on left side

B. Resident on back

C. Resident on right side

FIGURE I-9. Positions for rotating enema *(From Caldwell and Hegner,* Nursing Assistant, A Nursing Process Approach, *5th Edition, 1989, Delmar Publishers Inc.)*

5. Help resident assume left Sims' position and place bed protector under resident.
6. Insert lubricated tip 2–4 inches into rectum.
7. Allow about 300 ml of fluid to flow slowly into rectum.
8. Help resident to turn on back while you hold tube in place (Figure I-9).
9. Administer about 300 ml more of solution.
10. Holding tube in place, move solution can under resident's legs to other side of bed.
11. Assist resident to turn on right side and administer remaining solution.
12. Follow steps 16–29 for soapsuds enema.
 13. Perform procedure completion actions.

23. ENEMA, SOAPSUDS

Purpose of procedure: To remove feces and flatus from colon and rectum.

 1. Perform beginning procedure actions.
2. Assemble equipment:
   - Disposable enema equipment consisting of plastic container, tubing, clamp, and lubricant and packet of liquid soap.
   - Disposable gloves
   - Bedpan and cover or commode
   - Toilet tissue
   - Bed protector
   - Towel, soap, basin with warm water

NOTE: If disposable equipment is not available, you will need:
   - Funnel

- ■ Connecting tube
- ■ Graduate pitcher with warm, soapy water at 105°F
- ■ Pack of lubricant
- ■ Tubing and clamp
- ■ Rectal tube

3. In utility room:
    - ■ Connect tubing to solution container.
    - ■ Adjust clamp on tubing and snap shut.
    - ■ Fill container with warm water (105°F) to the 1000-ml line.
    - ■ Open packet of liquid soap and add to water in container.
    - ■ Use tip of tubing to gently mix solution.
    - ■ Run small amount of solution through tube to get rid of air and to warm tube.
    - ■ Lubricate tube and insert end of tube in lubricant packet or on paper towel. (Some kits have prelubricated tubes.)

4. Place chair at foot of bed and put covered bedpan on chair or position commode close to bed.

5. If resident will use bathroom or commode:
    - ■ Have resident's slippers and robe close by or help resident put them on before the enema.

6. Help resident assume left Sims' position and place bed protector under resident.

7. Put on gloves.

8. Expose only resident's buttocks by drawing bedding upward in one hand.

9. Separate buttocks and insert tube 2–4 inches into rectum.

10. Never force tube. If it cannot be inserted, report to nurse.
11. Open clamp and raise container 12 inches above level of anus (Figure I–10).
    ▪ Ask resident to take deep breaths to relax abdomen.
    ▪ If resident complains of cramping, clamp tube and wait until cramping stops.
    ▪ Then open tubing to continue fluid flow.
12. When enough solution has been given, clamp tubing.
13. Tell resident to hold breath while upper buttocks are raised and tube is gently withdrawn.

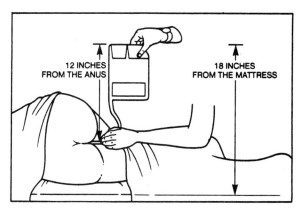

12 INCHES FROM THE ANUS

18 INCHES FROM THE MATTRESS

FIGURE I–10. Hang or hold container of soapsuds 12 inches from anus. *(From Caldwell and Hegner,* Assisting in Long-Term Care, *1988, Delmar Publishers Inc.)*

14. Wrap tubing in paper towel. Put it in disposable container.
15. Place resident on bedpan or assist to bathroom or commode.
16. Remove gloves.
17. If resident is on bedpan, raise head of bed and position for comfort.
18. Place toilet tissue and signal within reach of resident. If resident is in bathroom or on commode, stay nearby. Caution resident not to flush toilet.
19. When resident signals, remove bedpan or assist resident to return to bed.
20. Assist resident to clean perineal and rectal area if necessary. Put on gloves if resident needs help.
21. Remove bed protector.
22. Observe results of enema.
23. Flush toilet or cover bedpan or commode and empty contents according to facility policy.
24. Remove and discard gloves. Wash hands.
25. Assist resident to wash and dry hands.
26. Clean or dispose of equipment according to facility policy.

(**NOTE:** Many facilities clean disposable soapsuds enema kits to be used again by the same resident. If saved, clean according to facility policy and label kit with resident's name and room number. Store in bedside table or bathroom.)

➡ 27. Perform procedure completion actions.

24. HEARING AID, APPLYING

Purpose of procedure: To assist with insertion of hearing aid (Figure I-11).

1. Perform beginning procedure actions.
2. Assemble equipment:
   ■ Hearing aid
3. Check hearing aid to be sure batteries are working and tubing is not cracked.
4. Check resident's ear for wax buildup or any abnormalities.

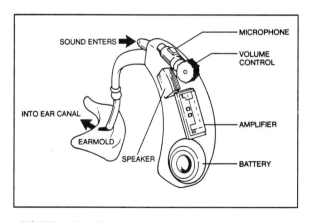

FIGURE I-11. Carefully position hearing aid behind ear. Ear mold fits into resident's ear canal. *(From Caldwell and Hegner, Assisting in Long-Term Care, 1988, Delmar Publishers Inc.)*

(**NOTE:** If resident complains that hearing aid hurts or doesn't fit properly, it may need to be refitted as ear structure changes with age. Notify nurse.)

   5. Handle aid carefully.
      ■ Do not drop it.
      ■ Do not allow it to get wet.
      ■ Store it carefully with switch in off position when it is not in use. Some aids should have batteries removed when being stored.
   6. Hand aid to resident so that you support the appliance as resident inserts earmold into ear canal.

 7. Perform procedure completion actions.

25. HEAT LAMP, APPLYING

Purpose of procedure: To provide a method of applying dry heat to increase blood supply to an area or to promote healing.

(**NOTE:** This procedure should be closely supervised by the nurse.)

   1. Perform beginning procedure actions.
   2. Assemble equipment:
      ■ Bath blanket
      ■ Tape measure
      ■ Heat lamp
   3. Position resident and drape with bath blanket so only area to be treated is exposed.

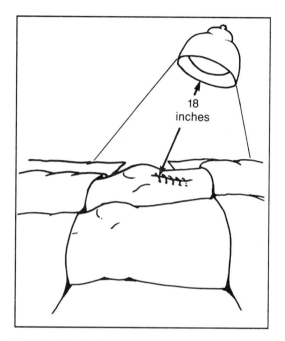

FIGURE I-12. Position heat lamp 18 inches from area being treated. *(From Caldwell and Hegner,* Nursing Assistant, A Nursing Process Approach, *5th Edition, 1989, Delmar Publishers Inc.)*

4. Position lamp at safe distance from resident.
   - Distance is determined by wattage of bulb.
   - A 40-watt bulb is usually used.
   - Light is positioned 18 inches from resident's body (Figure I-12).

5. Check distance with tape measure.

(**NOTE:** Residents must be cautioned not to move during treatment to make sure they do not come closer than 18 inches from heat source.)

6. Turn lamp on, noting time.
7. Check resident every five minutes. Carefully observe skin for signs of redness or burning.
8. Discontinue procedure after prescribed time.
9. Adjust bedding and remove drape. If procedure is to be repeated, fold and leave bath blanket in bedside table.
10. Perform procedure completion actions.

26. ICEBAG, APPLYING

Purpose of procedure: To provide a method of applying dry cold; to constrict blood vessels; to numb pain sensation; to slow inflammation or reduce itching.

1. Perform beginning procedure actions.
2. Assemble equipment:
    - Ice cap or collar
    - Cover (usually cotton)
    - Paper towels
    - Spoon or scoop
    - Ice cubes or crushed ice
3. Prepare ice cap or bag as follows:
    - If cubes are used, rinse in water to remove sharp edges.
    - Fill ice cap half full, using ice scoop or spoon. Avoid making bag too heavy (Figure I-13).
    - Expel air from bag by resting bag on table in horizontal position with top in place but not screwed on. Squeeze bag until air is removed.
    - Fasten top securely.
    - Test for leakage.
    - Wipe dry with paper towels and put bag in cotton cover.
4. Take equipment to bedside.
5. Apply icebag or collar to affected part with metal cap away from resident.

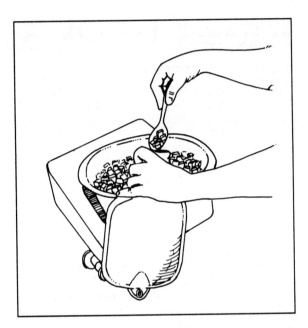

FIGURE I-13. Fill ice bag half full and expel air. *(From Caldwell and Hegner,* Nursing Assistant, A Nursing Process Approach, *5th Edition, 1989, Delmar Publishers Inc.)*

   6. Refill bag before ice is melted.
   7. Check skin area with each application. Report to nurse immediately if skin is discolored or white or if resident reports skin is numb.
   8. Perform procedure completion actions.

(**NOTE:** If frozen gel pak is available, take from freezer and proceed as with ice bag.)

27. ILEOSTOMY, ROUTINE CARE WITH RESIDENT IN BED

Purpose of procedure: To clean stoma site, preventing skin irritation and breakdown; to prevent odors (Figure I-14).

1. Perform beginning procedure actions.
2. Assemble equipment:
   - Basin of warm water
   - Bed protector
   - Bath blanket
   - Bedpan/cover

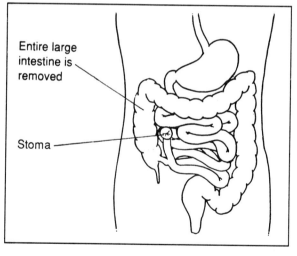

Entire large intestine is removed

Stoma

FIGURE I-14. An ileostomy brings a section of ileum (small intestine) through abdominal wall. *(From Caldwell and Hegner, Nursing Assistant, A Nursing Process Approach, 5th Edition, 1989, Delmar Publishers Inc.)*

- Disposable gloves
- Fresh appliance and belt
- Clamp for appliance
- Prescribed solvent/dropper
- Cotton balls
- Deodorant (if permitted)
- Soap or cleansing agent
- Karaya ring
- 4 × 4 Gauze squares
- Toilet tissue
- Paper towels

3. Raise opposite siderail for safety. Elevate head of bed and assist resident to turn on side toward you.
4. Replace top bedding with bath blanket.
5. Place bed protector under resident.
6. Put on disposable gloves.
7. Place bedpan or bed protector against resident.
8. Place end of ileostomy bag in bedpan. Open clamp and allow to drain. Note amount and character of drainage.
9. Wipe end of drainage sheath with toilet paper and move out of drainage. Place tissue in bedpan and cover.
10. Disconnect belt from appliance and remove from resident. Place on paper towels.
11. With dropper, apply small amount of solvent around ring of appliance to loosen it. Wait a few minutes and do not force appliance free.
12. Cover stoma with gauze.
    - Carefully inspect skin area around stoma.

- ∎ If area is irritated or skin is broken, cover resident with bath blanket. Raise side-rails. Lower bed.

13. Remove and discard gloves. Wash your hands and report to nurse for instructions.

14. Gently cleanse area around stoma with cotton balls. Use soap or other cleansing agent. Gently pat dry.

15. Remove gauze from stoma and place in paper towels.

16. If appliance is used with Karaya ring, moisten ring, allow it to become sticky and apply to stoma. (If appliance used paper-covered adhesive strip around stoma opening, remove paper and apply around stoma.)

17. Clamp appliance bag, add deodorant (if allowed), and apply to ring.

18. Adjust a clean belt in position around resident and connect to appliance.

19. Remove covered bedpan and place on chair on paper towels.

20. Remove bed protector and disposable gloves and place on bedpan. Check bottom bedding and change if wet.

21. Replace bath blanket with top bedding.

22. Gather soiled materials and bedpan.
    - ∎ Take to utility room.
    - ∎ Dispose of according to facility policy.
    - ∎ If belt and bag are reusable, wash and allow to dry.

23. Empty, wash, and dry bedpan and return to resident's unit.

24. Perform procedure completion actions.

28. ILEOSTOMY, ROUTINE CARE WITH RESIDENT IN BATHROOM

Purpose of procedure: To clean stoma site, preventing skin irritation and breakdown; to prevent odors.

1. Perform beginning procedure actions.
2. Assemble equipment:
   - Disposable gloves
   - Fresh appliance and belt
   - Bath blanket
   - Clamp for appliance
   - Cotton balls
   - Solvent/dropper
   - Deodorant
   - Soap and cleansing agent
   - Karaya ring
   - 4 × 4 Gauze squares
   - Paper towels
3. Take equipment to resident's bathroom.
4. Assist resident into robe and slippers.
5. Assist resident into bathroom and position on toilet (Figure I-15).
6. Place bath blanket over resident's legs. Raise gown and roll at waist, exposing appliance. Instruct resident to separate legs.
7. Put on gloves. Open ileostomy appliance, directing drainage into toilet. Note character and amount of drainage.
8. With dropper, apply small amount of solvent around Karaya gum ring to loosen from skin. Do not force from skin.
9. Cover stoma with gauze sponge to collect drainage.

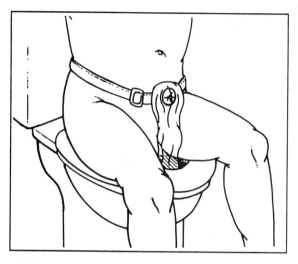

FIGURE I-15. Direct end of drainage bag into toilet. *(From Caldwell and Hegner,* Nursing Assistant, A Nursing Process Approach, *5th Edition, 1989, Delmar Publishers Inc.)*

10. With cotton balls, cleanse area around stoma with warm water and soap or cleansing agent. (If skin is broken, report to nurse for instructions.) Pat area dry.
11. Remove gauze from stoma and place in paper towels.
12. If appliance is used with Karaya ring, moisten ring, allow to become sticky and apply to stoma. (If appliance uses paper-covered adhesive strip around stoma opening, remove paper and apply around stoma.)
13. Clamp appliance bag and apply to ring.

14. Remove gloves, adjust clean belt in position around resident and connect to appliance.
15. Remove bath blanket and assist resident to wash hands and dress or return to bed.
16. Clean resident's bathroom. Wash belt and appliance, if reusable, and allow to dry.
17. Perform procedure completion actions.

29. INTAKE (Fluid), MEASURING AND RECORDING (See also, Output)

Purpose of procedure: To provide accurate records of fluid intake for residents who are dehydrated; receiving intravenous fluids; are losing fluids through perspiration, vomitus or stool; who have had recent surgery; or who are retaining body fluids.

1. Perform beginning procedure actions.
2. Assemble equipment:
   - Intake and output record at bedside
   - Chart with fluid content of containers used at your facility
   - Pen for recording
   - Resident's meal tray, water pitcher, and/ or between meal nourishment dishes
3. Oral fluid intake is recorded for these items taken by resident:
   - Ice chips, water, juices.
   - Carbonated beverages, coffee, tea.
   - Soups, Jell-O, ice cream, sherbet, Popsicles.
   - Any food that becomes liquid at room temperature.
4. Record all fluid intake that is consumed at meals and between meals.

5. Intravenous fluids and tube feedings are also recorded as intake. The nurse assumes responsibility for recording these items.

6. Fluid intake is recorded as milliliters (ml), which are the same as cubic centimeters (cc).

7. The total is recorded at the end of each shift and the end of twenty-four hours.

8. To record intake:
   - Look at chart to see how many ml the container holds when it is full (Figure I-16).
   - Look at container that resident drank from to see how much is gone.

Drinking glass = 6 oz = 180 cc   Jell-O = 4 oz = 120 cc
Styrofoam cup = 6 oz = 180 cc   Ice cream cup = 5 oz = 150 cc
Juice glass (small) = 4 oz = 120 cc   Creamer = 1 oz = 30 cc
Juice glass (large) = 8 oz = 240 cc
Full water
   pitcher (1 qt) = 32 oz = 960 cc   **Abbreviations**
Coffee or tea pot = 10 oz = 300 cc
Coffee cup = 5 oz = 150 cc   oz = ounce = 30 cc
Milk carton = 8 oz = 240 cc   pt = pint = 16 oz = 480/500 cc
Soup bowl (small) = 6 oz = 180 cc   qt = quart = 32 oz = 960/1000 cc
Soup bowl (large) = 10 oz = 300 cc   gal = gallon = 128 oz = 3840/4000 cc

Residents may not finish all fluids furnished to them. Estimate how much fluid has actually been taken and record the amount. For instance, the resident is given 8 ounces of milk but drinks only 4 ounces. Therefore, record intake of 120 cc.

FIGURE I-16. Average container amounts *(From Caldwell and Hegner,* Assisting in Long-Term Care, *5th Edition, 1989, Delmar Publishers Inc.)*

■ For example, if a cup holds 240 ml when full and the resident has consumed one-third of fluid in the container, then resident's intake is 80 ml

(1/3 × 240 = 80).

■ *Always record amount that is gone from containers.*

9. Do this for each container and record intake from each container on intake and output record.

■ In some facilities, the total amount of ml from the meal is recorded on the record instead of amounts from each separate item that was consumed.

■ In this case, calculate intake from each container, add these amounts together, and enter this figure on intake record.

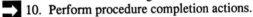 10. Perform procedure completion actions.

30. ISOLATION PROCEDURES

Remember that frequent and thorough handwashing is the most important procedure for preventing the spread of disease. Isolation procedures include using personal protective equipment to further decrease the risk of spreading infectious disease. (See Section D, Infection Control, for additional information.)

a. Caring for Linens in Isolation Unit

Purpose of procedure: To avoid contaminating linens needlessly; to avoid spreading microorganisms through careless handling of soiled linens.

1. Bring clean linen to unit as needed.

2. Handle soiled linen as little as possible.
3. Place soiled linens in leakproof laundry bag inside isolation unit.
4. Bag should be labeled and identified by color code.
5. Double-bag soiled linens if required.
6. Secure bag and route soiled linen according to facility policy.

b. Double-bagging

Purpose of procedure: To prevent the spread of microorganisms by bagging soiled linens or other contaminated items, twice.

(NOTE: Some facilities place soiled linens in dissolvable bags, inside the unit. This bag containing the soiled linens is then placed in a canvas bag during the double-bagging procedure. Remember that dissolvable bags may begin to disintegrate when wet.)

1. Perform beginning procedure actions.
2. Assemble equipment:
   ■ Clean bag for linens or items to be double-bagged
3. You will need another assistant to help you with this procedure.
4. A "clean" person stands outside the unit while the other person is inside the unit.
5. Person inside the unit places item in isolation bag and secures bag with tie.
6. Clean person on outside of unit holds cuffed plastic bag over hands (to avoid contaminating hands) to receive bagged item.

7. Clean person tightly secures top of plastic bag.
8. Clean person removes double-bagged item. Disposable items are routed as infectious waste.

 9. Perform procedure completion actions.

c. Gloves, Putting On

Purpose of procedure: To provide additional protection to the health care provider and to prevent the spread of microorganisms to residents.

(**NOTE:** Personal protective equipment or barrier equipment refers to gloves, gowns, masks, and other items worn to protect the health care provider against microorganisms.)

1. Perform beginning procedure actions.
2. Assemble equipment:
   ■ Disposable gloves in correct size
3. Wash hands.
4. If gown is required, put on gloves after gown is put on.
5. Pick up glove by the cuff with right hand and place it on your left hand.
6. Repeat with glove for right hand.
7. Interlace fingers to adjust gloves on hands.
8. Remember when using gloves:
   ■ Wash hands before and after using gloves.
   ■ Remove gloves if they tear or become heavily soiled. Wash hands and put on a new pair.
   ■ Gloves are used whenever there is the possibility of contact with body fluids or blood.

- When wearing gloves for universal precautions, change gloves between residents and wash hands.
- Discard gloves immediately after removing, in appropriate waste receptacle.

 9. Perform procedure completion actions.

d. Gown, Putting On

Purpose of procedure: To prevent contaminating the health care provider's uniform.

(NOTE: To be effective, a gown should have long sleeves, be long enough to cover the uniform, and big enough to overlap in the back. Gowns should be waterproof.)

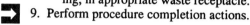 1. Perform beginning procedure actions.
2. Assemble equipment:
   - Clean gown
   - Paper towel
3. Remove wristwatch, place it on clean side of open paper towel.
4. Wash hands.
5. Put on gown by slipping arms into sleeves.
6. Slip fingers under inside neckband and grasp ties in back. Secure neckband.
7. Reach behind and overlap edges of gown. Secure waist ties.
8. Take watch into isolation unit, leaving it on paper towel so it doesn't have to be touched.
9. Remember when using gowns:
   - A disposable gown is only worn once and is then discarded as infectious waste.
   - A cloth, reusable gown is only worn once and is then handled as contaminated linen.

■ Perform all procedures in the unit at one
time to avoid unnecessary waste of gowns.

 10. Perform procedure completion actions.

e. Mask, Putting On

Purpose of procedure: To prevent the spread of microorganisms through the respiratory tract.

 1. Perform beginning procedure actions.
2. Assemble equipment:
    ■ Mask
3. If gown and gloves are needed, the mask goes on first.
4. Adjust mask over nose and mouth.
5. Tie top strings of mask first, then bottom strings.
6. Replace mask if it becomes moist during procedure.
 7. Perform procedure completion actions.

f. Removing Contaminated Gown, Gloves, and Mask

Purpose of procedure: To remove contaminated personal protective equipment without contamination of uniform or self.

1. Perform beginning procedure actions.
2. Assemble equipment:
    ■ Waste receptacle for disposable items
    ■ Waste receptacle for gown if it is not disposable
    ■ Paper towels
    ■ Soap and water for handwashing

3. Remove gloves first:
   - Grasp cuff of left hand glove with right hand and bring cuff down over glove, turning glove inside out.
   - Repeat with other glove.
   - Discard in appropriate waste receptacle.
4. Undo waist ties of gown.
5. Turn faucets on with clean paper towel. Discard towel.
6. Wash hands and dry with clean paper towel.
7. Hold clean, dry paper towel to turn off faucet.
8. Undo mask:
   - Bottom ties first, then top ties.
   - Holding top ties, dispose of mask in appropriate waste receptacle.
9. Undo neck ties and loosen gown at shoulders.
10. Slip fingers of right hand inside left cuff without touching outside of gown. Pull gown down over left hand (Figure I-17A).
11. With gown-covered left hand, pull gown down over right hand (Figure I-17B).
12. Fold gown with contaminated side inward. Roll and dispose of in appropriate receptacle (Figure I-17C).
13. Wash hands.
14. Remove watch from clean side of paper towel. Hold clean side of paper towel, dispose of towel in wastepaper receptacle.
15. Perform procedure completion actions.

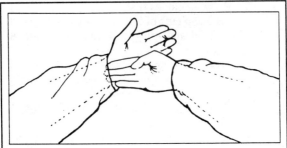

A. Slip fingers of right hand inside left cuff of gown and pull gown, as shown, over left hand. Do not touch outside of gown with right hand.

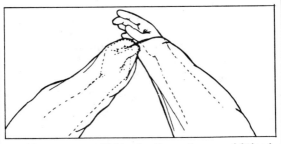

B. Using gown-covered left hand, pull gown down over right hand.

FIGURE I-17. Removing contaminated gown *(From Caldwell and Hegner,* Nursing Assistant, A Nursing Process Approach, *5th Edition, 1989, Delmar Publishers Inc.)*

g. Specimen Collection from Resident in Isolation Unit

Purpose of procedure: To send specimen to laboratory without spreading microorganisms from resident's unit.

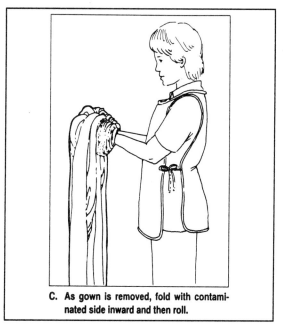

C. As gown is removed, fold with contaminated side inward and then roll.

FIGURE I-17. Removing contaminated gown (continued) *(From Caldwell and Hegner,* Nursing Assistant, A Nursing Process Approach, *5th Edition, 1989, Delmar Publishers Inc.)*

 1. Perform beginning procedure actions.
2. Assemble equipment.
   - ■ Clean specimen container and cover
   - ■ Paper towel
   - ■ Gloves
   - ■ Plastic bag for specimen container

3. Bring clean specimen container and cover into unit. Place them on clean paper towel.
4. Put on gloves. (Put on gown and mask, if required.) Place specimen in container without touching container.
5. Cover specimen and label.
6. Remove and discard gloves. Wash your hands.
7. Using paper towel, pick up specimen container and place in plastic bag. Have specimen transported to laboratory.

h. Transferring Nondisposable Equipment Outside of Isolation Unit

Purpose of procedure: To remove nondisposable equipment from isolation unit without spreading microorganisms.

1. Perform beginning procedure actions.
2. Assemble equipment:
   ■ Equipment to be removed from unit
   ■ Gloves, gown, mask if required
   ■ Bags for double-bagging if required
3. Equipment that requires processing may be double-bagged to be sterilized.
4. Some equipment may be terminally cleaned with disinfectant in the resident's unit.
5. Perform procedure completion actions when finished.

i. Transporting Resident in Isolation

Purpose of procedure: To remove resident to another part of the facility without spreading microorganisms.

1. Perform beginning procedure actions.
2. Assemble equipment:
    ■ Transport vehicle (stretcher or wheel-chair)
    ■ Clean sheet
    ■ Gown, mask, gloves if required
3. Notify receiving department that resident from isolation is being transported to their department.
4. Cover transport vehicle with clean sheet and wheel vehicle into room.
5. Identify resident and explain what you plan to do and how resident can assist you.
6. If required, put on appropriate barriers: gown, mask, gloves.
7. Assist resident into transport vehicle.
8. Put mask on resident if required.
9. Wrap resident in sheet if required.
10. Remove your gown and other barriers as you leave unit.
11. Upon return from other department, return resident to unit. Follow barrier technique as required and return resident to bed.
12. Remove sheet from transport vehicle and deposit in isolation laundry hamper.
13. Perform procedure completion actions.

31. KETODIASTIX®: TESTING URINE FOR SUGAR AND KETONES (Acetone)

Purpose of procedure: To determine the presence and amount of sugar and acetone in the urine of diabetic residents.

1. Perform beginning procedure actions.
2. Assemble equipment:
   - Sample of freshly voided urine in container
   - Ketodiastix® reagent strips
   - Watch with second hand
3. Ask resident to empty bladder about one hour before test is to be done.
4. Test this urine immediately in case resident is unable to void later.
5. Ask resident to empty bladder again at the time the test is to be done.
6. If resident is able to urinate, test this specimen and discard earlier one.
7. Dip end of Ketodiastix® strip (end with reagent areas) into the urine.
8. Remove strip, tap it gently on edge of urine container and hold strip horizontally.
9. After 15 seconds, compare buff-colored strip with color chart on bottle label for ketones.

Match it as closely as possible to one color on the chart.

10. At the end of another 15 seconds (a total of 30 seconds from starting time), check the blue-colored strip with color chart on bottle label for sugar (glucose). Match it as closely as possible to one color on the chart.

11. Do not discard specimen until you are sure of the results. If there is a question, retest specimen with a fresh reagent strip or report to the nurse for further instructions.

12. When testing is completed, discard urine specimen according to facility policy.

13. Perform procedure completion actions.

L

---

32. LOG ROLLING

Purpose of procedure: To keep resident's spinal column straight while turning the resident. This is performed following spinal surgery or injury to spinal cord or vertebral column.

1. Perform beginning procedure actions.
2. Assemble equipment:
   - Turning sheet if one will be used
   - Pillow
3. Get another assistant to help you.
4. Elevate head of bed to comfortable working position and lock wheels.
5. Lower siderail on side opposite to which resident will be turned. Both assistants work from same side of bed.
6. One assistant places hands under resident's head and shoulder.
   - Second person places hands under resident's hips and legs.
   - Move resident as a unit toward you.
7. Place a pillow lengthwise between resident's legs. Fold resident's arms over his/her chest.
8. Raise siderail and check for security.
9. Go to opposite side of bed and lower rail.
10. Turning resident to side may be done by:
    - Using a turning sheet that has been previously placed under resident.

11. Reach over resident, grasping and rolling turning sheet toward resident.
12. One assistant should be positioned beside resident to keep resident's shoulders and hips straight.
13. Second assistant should be positioned to keep resident's thighs and lower legs straight.
    ■ If a turning sheet is not in position, first assistant should position hands on resident's far thigh and lower leg.
14. At a specified signal, the resident is drawn toward both assistants in a single movement, keeping resident's spine, head, and legs in straight position.
15. Place additional pillows behind resident to maintain position. A small pillow or folded bath blanket may be permitted under resident's head and neck. Leave a pillow between resident's legs. Position small pillows or folded towels to support resident's arms.

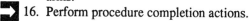

16. Perform procedure completion actions.

════ M ════

33. MECHANICAL LIFT TO TRANSFER RESIDENT

Purpose of procedure: To transfer resident in and out of bed. This procedure is usually used for heavy residents who have little or no weight bearing ability.

(**NOTE:** Check slings, chains, and straps for frayed areas or poorly closing clasps. Do not use defective equipment. Report need of repair and obtain safe equipment.)

1. Perform beginning procedure actions.
2. Assemble equipment:
   - Mechanical lift
   - Sling

(**NOTE:** Two people should perform these procedures to ensure safety of the resident.)

3. Place wheelchair or other chair at right angle to foot of bed, facing head. Lock wheelchair.
4. Elevate bed to comfortable working height. Lock wheels of bed. Lower nearest siderail. Roll resident toward you.
5. Position slings beneath resident's body behind shoulder, thighs, and buttocks. Be sure sling is smooth.

6. Roll resident back onto sling and position properly. If sling has inserts for metal bars, insert these now.

7. Attach suspension straps to sling. Check fasteners for security.

(**NOTE:** Be sure that right end of strap or chain is hooked to right place on sling. Always hook straps from inside to out.)

8. Position lift frame over bed with base legs in maximum open position and lock.

9. Attach suspension straps or chain to frame. Position resident's arms inside straps.

10. Secure straps or chains if necessary.

11. Talk to resident while slowly lifting resident free of bed.

12. Guide lift away from bed.

13. Position resident close to chair or wheelchair. Make sure wheels of wheelchair are locked.

14. Slowly lower resident into chair or wheelchair. Pay attention to position of resident's feet and hands.

15. Unhook suspension straps or chains and remove lift.

16. If resident is in chair, sling can remain underneath resident so it is in position for transfer back to bed. If sling has metal bars, remove these and make sure sling is smooth and wrinkle free.

17. If resident has returned to bed, remove sling.

(NOTE: The method for raising and lowering lift and for moving base legs varies for different types of equipment. Please read manufacturer's directions and practice using equipment *before* using it with residents.)

 18. Perform procedure completion actions.

34. MOIST COMPRESS, APPLYING

Purpose of procedure: To apply moist heat or moist cold to an area of resident's body.

 1. Perform beginning procedure actions.
2. Assemble equipment:
    - Disposable gloves
    - Syringe to keep dressings moist
    - Bed protector
    - Compresses
    - Bath thermometer
    - Binder or towel
    - Pins or bandage
    - Basin with prescribed solution at temperature ordered
3. Bring equipment to bedside.
4. Expose only area to be treated.
5. Protect bed and resident's clothing with bed protector.
6. Put on gloves.

7. Moisten compresses; remove excess liquid and apply to treatment area.
8. Remove and discard gloves.
9. Secure compresses with bandage or binder. Compress must be in contact with skin.
10. Wash hands.
11. Help resident maintain comfortable position throughout treatment.
12. Unscreen unit. Leave unit neat and tidy with signal cord within easy reach.
13. Maintain proper temperature and moisture.
    ■ If compresses are to be kept warm, a warm water bottle or Aquamatic K Pad® may be applied.
    ■ If compresses are to be kept cool, an ice bag may be applied.
    ■ A syringe may be used to apply solution to keep compresses wet.
14. Remove compresses when ordered. Change as ordered. Check skin several times each day.
15. Discard compresses.
16. Perform procedure completion actions.

35. OUTPUT (Fluid), MEASURING AND RECORDING (See also, Intake)

Purpose of procedure: To monitor fluid output of residents who are dehydrated; retaining fluids; receiving intravenous therapy; have indwelling catheters; are losing body fluids through perspiration, vomiting, loose stools or urine.

1. Perform beginning procedure actions.
2. Assemble equipment:
   - Graduate pitcher
   - Pen for recording
   - Disposable gloves
3. Put on disposable gloves.
4. Drain urine from catheter drainage bag into graduate according to procedure and take covered container to resident's bathroom or utility room. If resident uses bedpan or urinal, cover and take to resident's bathroom or utility room.
5. Pour urine from bedpan or urinal into graduate. Hold graduate at eye level and note amount.
   - If resident uses toilet, a hat-shaped specimen container is placed on toilet. Measure, empty, and rinse container.

6. Record amount immediately under output column on intake and output record.
7. All output is recorded and includes:
   - Urine
   - Vomitus (emesis)
   - Drainage from wound or stomach
   - Liquid stool
   - Blood loss (measured by marking dressings or measuring amount in hemovac container)
   - Perspiration (estimated amount: small, moderate, or excessive)
8. If specimens are required, save and send to laboratory as facility policy indicates. If specimen is not needed, discard fluids in bedpan hopper or toilet.
9. Clean graduate and other utensils according to facility policy.
10. Remove gloves and discard. Wash hands.
11. Perform procedure completion actions.

(**NOTE:** For incontinent residents, incontinent pads may be weighed before placing them under resident and again when they are changed. Subtract the difference to find the amount of urine or stool in the pad.)

36. POSITIONING RESIDENT IN BED

Purpose of procedure: To help resident feel more comfortable; to relieve strain and joint stiffness; to help body function more efficiently; to prevent complications such as contractures and pressure sores.

1. Perform beginning procedure actions.
2. Assemble equipment:
     ■ Extra pillows (folded mattress pads, folded bath blankets, and towels can be used if there are not enough pillows)
     ■ Handrolls if required
     ■ Trochanter rolls if required (these can be formed from bath blankets)
3. Remember these principles for positioning:
     ■ Always place resident in good body alignment before positioning. Move resident to head of bed and/or to side of bed if necessary. Use a turning sheet for these procedures.
     ■ Place joints in neutral position, avoiding flexion if possible. Try to avoid:
        — Flexion or hyperextension of the neck
        — Adduction of shoulders
        — Adduction and external rotation of hips
        — Plantar flexion of ankle
     ■ Use handrolls only if instructed to do so by nurse. Handrolls should be firm and smooth. This keeps the hands from flexing too much. A folded washcloth should never be used for this purpose.

- Use a footboard only if instructed to do so. Make sure covers are loose over resident's feet.
- When resident is in side-lying position (lateral recumbent), support upper wrist and hand, ankle and foot. Position resident so body weight is not directly on shoulder and hip.
- A resident's position should be changed at least every two hours.
- When changing position, always check resident's skin for signs of redness or breakdown.

 4. Perform beginning procedure actions before changing resident's position.
  5. Positions:
   - Horizontal Recumbent (supine or back-lying) (Figure I-18).
   — Bed is flat with resident on back.

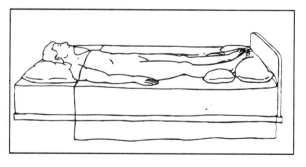

FIGURE I-18. Horizontal recumbent position (supine or back-lying) *(From Caldwell and Hegner,* Nursing Assistant, A Nursing Process Approach, *5th Edition, 1989, Delmar Publishers Inc.)*

— Pillow is placed under head for comfort. Make sure it extends down below shoulders.
— Arms are extended and supported by small pillows extending from elbows to ends of fingers.
— A small pillow, rolled towel, or trochanter roll is placed along side and tucked under resident's hip joints to prevent external hip rotation.
— Place a pillow against resident's feet.
— Place small pillow or folded pad under legs extending from knees to ankles.

■ Prone Position (face-lying) (Figure I-19)

(NOTE: Most elderly people are not able or do not like to be in this position. Use this position only when instructed to do so by the nurse. Before turning a dependent person prone,

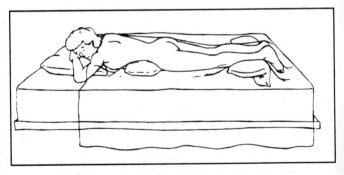

FIGURE I-19. Prone position (face-lying) *(From Caldwell and Hegner,* Nursing Assistant, A Nursing Process Approach, *5th Edition, 1989, Delmar Publishers Inc.)*

make sure resident's arms are straight down at sides to avoid injury while turning. Never leave an older person in this position for more than 15–20 minutes.)

— Resident is on abdomen and spine is straight with face turned to either side.

— Legs are extended. Arms are flexed and brought up to either side of head.

— A small pillow can be placed under abdomen, especially for females as this reduces pressure against breasts. An alternative method is to roll a towel and place it under shoulders to reduce pressure.

— Place another pillow under lower legs to prevent pressure on toes.

— Resident may also be moved to foot of bed so feet extend over mattress. This is an alternative method for preventing pressure on toes.

■ Semi-Fowler's Position (Figure I-20)

— Resident is on back with head of bed elevated 30 degrees. Fowler's position is 45–60 degrees and high Fowler's is 90 degrees.

— Place one, two, or three pillows to support head and shoulders.

— Knees may be slightly flexed and supported with small pillows.

— Pillows may be placed under each arm from elbows to fingertips to support shoulders.

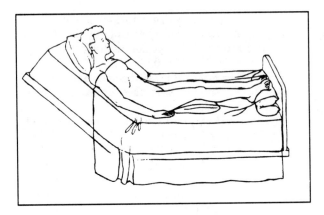

FIGURE I-20. Semi-Fowler's position *(From Caldwell and Hegner, Nursing Assistant, A Nursing Process Approach, 5th Edition, 1989, Delmar Publishers Inc.)*

    — Place pillow against feet.
- Sims' Position. (This position is usually used only for examination or administration of enemas.)
- Lateral Recumbent Position (side-lying).
  - Turn resident on either right or left side. Be sure resident will not be lying too close to either siderail when you are finished.
  - Spine should be straight and in alignment with bed.
  - Place pillow(s) under top arm with arm slightly flexed and in front of resident. Shoulder, elbow, and wrist should be supported to same height.

- Place pillow(s) between legs with top leg slightly flexed and forward. Hip, knee, and ankle should be supported to same height.
- Bottom arm is flexed with palm of hand facing up.
- Place pillows behind resident's back, if necessary, to maintain position.

 6. Perform procedure completion actions.

37. POSITIONING RESIDENT IN A CHAIR

Purpose of procedure: To reduce pressure to coccyx (tailbone); to maintain body alignment; to increase resident's comfort.

(**NOTE:** Wheelchairs are intended to be used for transport. They are not appropriate chairs for long periods of sitting. If resident must remain in wheelchair for an extended period of time, assist resident to do pressure relieving exercises.)

 1. Perform beginning procedure actions.
2. Assemble equipment:
    ■ Pillows or folded towels as needed
3. Chair position:
    ■ Head and spine are erect in body alignment.
    ■ Arms rest on arms of chair or in resident's lap. If shoulders are pushed upward, resident needs a cushion under buttocks to allow shoulders to assume natural position.

■ If shoulders are hanging, pillows can be placed under resident's lower arms.
■ Back and buttocks are up against back of chair.
■ Feet are flat on floor. Use footstool if resident's legs are too short to reach floor.
■ Use pillows or postural supports to maintain position. (Postural supports are commercially purchased items. Follow manufacturer's instructions for application.)
■ Small pillow or folded towel can be placed at small of back.
■ Do not permit back of knees to rest against chair.

4. Wheelchair exercises:
   ■ Leaning to ease pressure.
     — Make sure wheels of chair are locked.
     — Have resident lean forward with chest over knees. (Don't let resident fall forward out of chair.)
     — Have resident lean from side to side, getting as much weight as possible off each hip.
   ■ Wheelchair pushups:
     — Make sure wheels of chair are locked.
     — Foot pedals should be in up position or off the wheelchair.
     — Tell resident to place palms of hands on arms of chair and to flex elbows.
     — Have resident lean forward, put feet back, and spread knees.
     — Now have resident lift buttocks off chair by pushing down with hands and straightening knees.

5. To move a sliding resident back and up in a wheelchair:
   - Get another assistant to help you. One stands in back of the wheelchair and one stands in front of resident.
   - Make sure wheels of chair are locked.
   - Both assistants separate their feet, bend knees, and hips and keep backs straight.
   - Assistant in back places both arms around resident's waist, crossing her/his own arms in front of resident's waist.
   - Assistant in front places both arms around resident's knees.
   - On count of three, both assistants lift and raise resident up and back in chair.
   - Lift sheets can be placed in seats of chairs for residents who are very frail or very heavy.

 6. Perform procedure completion actions.

38. POSTMORTEM CARE

Purpose of procedure: To prepare resident's deceased body for transfer to the mortuary.

1. Perform beginning procedure actions.
2. Assemble equipment:
   - Shroud or clean sheet
   - Basin with warm water
   - Washcloth
   - Towels
   - Disposable gloves
   - Identification cards (3)
   - Cotton

- Bandages
- Pads as needed

3. Nurse should remove appliances and body tubes.
4. Work quickly and quietly, maintaining an attitude of respect.
5. Place the body on the back with head and shoulders elevated on pillow.
   - Close eyes by grasping eyelashes. Place moistened cotton ball on each eye if lids do not remain shut.
   - Replace dentures in resident's mouth. Replace artificial eye if resident has one.
   - Jaw may need to be secured with light bandaging. Place a pad beneath the bandage to avoid leaving marks.
6. Bathe as necessary. Remove soiled dressings and replace with new ones. Groom hair.
7. Pad between ankles and knees with cotton and tie lightly.
8. Prepare body for family viewing:
   - Place disposable pad underneath buttocks.
   - Put clean gown on resident.
   - Cover body to shoulders with sheet.
   - Make sure room is neat and tidy.
   - Allow family to be with resident in private.
9. Put shroud on resident after family leaves.
10. Collect all belongings and check against admission list. Wrap properly and label. Valuables remain locked up until a relative signs for them.

11. Fill out identification cards and fasten according to facility policy.
12. Transport body to morgue on a gurney according to facility policy.

(**NOTE:** In some facilities, the body is left in the room until the funeral director arrives to remove the body to the funeral home.)

 13. Perform procedure completion actions.

39. PRESSURE SORE PREVENTION

Purpose of procedure: To prevent skin breakdown resulting from pressure.

 1. Perform beginning procedure actions.
2. Assemble equipment:
    - Clean linens as needed
    - Pillows and other positioning devices as needed
    - Basin of warm water about 105°F
    - Soap in soapdish
    - Towel and washcloth
    - Lotion
    - Gloves if needed
3. Reposition resident regularly, at least every two hours.
    - Always use a turning sheet to move resident in bed to avoid shearing the skin.
    - Inspect skin for signs of redness or breakdown (Figure I-21).
    - Teach residents to do wheelchair pushups to relieve pressure.

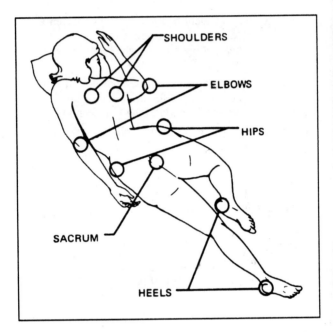

FIGURE I-21. Check these sites at least daily for signs of redness or skin breakdown. *(From Caldwell and Hegner,* Nursing Assistant, A Nursing Process Approach, *5th Edition, 1989, Delmar Publishers Inc.)*

4. Wash, rinse, and dry resident's back with bath, with AM and PM care, and as indicated by care plan.
5. Give lotion backrub each time back is washed.

- ■ Do not use alcohol as it is very drying.
- ■ Massage around reddened areas frequently but do not rub directly on top of reddened area.
- ■ Do not use lotion on broken skin areas.
- ■ If powder is used, apply sparingly. It can be abrasive if overused.

6. For incontinent residents, follow Steps 3–5 each time resident is incontinent. Use gloves. Immediately remove feces and urine from skin.
   - ■ Change linens and keep linen dry and free from wrinkles, crumbs, and other objects.

7. Maintain adequate food and fluid intake. Some residents may receive high protein nutritional supplements to prevent pressure sores.

8. Check for improperly fitting braces, restraints, or clothing.

9. Special mattresses, heel pads, or elbow pads may be used for residents at risk for pressure sores.

10. Perform range of motion exercises at least twice each day.

11. If resident develops a pressure sore, there are many modes of treatment. It is the physician's responsibility to order a specific treatment. It is the nurse's responsibility to perform the treatment.

12. Perform procedure completion actions.

■ **R** ■

40. RANGE OF MOTION EXERCISES (Passive)

Purpose of procedure: To provide exercise for a dependent resident; to prevent joint stiffness and contractures; to stimulate circulation and muscles.

1. Perform beginning procedure actions.
2. Assemble equipment:
   - Bath blanket
3. Encourage resident to do active or active assistive movements as you hold extremity.
4. Guidelines to remember when doing passive range of motion:
   - Do not attempt to passively move resident's neck.
   - Move each joint to full range unless orders state otherwise. This may be limited with elderly residents. Avoid causing pain.
   - Do each motion slowly, smoothly, and gently.
   - Hold extremities gently but firmly with the palms of your hands.
   - Do each movement at least five or six times.
   - These exercises are most effective when resident is in bed rather than in chair.
   - Do all movements of upper and lower extremity on one side and then move to other side of bed.
5. Cover resident with bath blanket and then move top covers to foot of bed. Place

resident's near arm on top of blanket and
begin with shoulder movements.

6. Shoulder movements
   - ■ Supporting elbow and wrist, exercise
     shoulder joint nearest you:
     — Bring entire arm out at right angle to
       body (abduction), and
     — Return arm to position parallel with
       body (adduction).
   - ■ With shoulder in adduction, flex elbow
     and raise entire arm over head (flexion).
     — Bring arm down parallel to body (ex-
       tension).
   - ■ With arm parallel to body, bring arm up
     and cross it over chest (horizontal adduc-
     tion), and then
     — Bring arm back so elbow is parallel to
       shoulder (horizontal abduction).
   - ■ With elbow parallel to shoulder, place
     forearm in up position with palm of hand
     up (external rotation).
     — Bring forearm down with elbow and
       shoulder remaining stationary (inter-
       nal rotation).

7. Elbow movements
   - ■ With arm parallel to body and palm up,
     bend elbow (flexion).
     — Return arm to position parallel to body
       and palm up (extension).
   - ■ Place your hand in resident's hand as if to
     shake hands. Turn resident's hand with
     yours so palm is down (pronation), and
     then

— Turn resident's hand with yours so resident's palm is up (supination).

8. Wrist movements
   ■ Supporting resident's forearm, bend wrist forward (flexion), and then
      — Straighten wrist out (extension), and then
      — Bend wrist backward carefully (hyperextension).
   ■ Supporting resident's forearm and wrist, move hand toward little finger side (ulnar deviation), and then
      — Toward thumb side (radial deviation).

9. Fingers and thumb
   ■ Curl fingers together (flexion), and then
      — Straighten each finger out (extension).
   ■ Move each finger, in turn, away from middle finger (abduction), and then
      — Toward the middle finger (adduction).
   ■ Repeat these movements with thumb.
   ■ Touch thumb to base of little finger and then to each fingertip (opposition).

10. Cover resident's arm and rearrange bath blanket just enough to expose leg. Face foot of bed.

11. Hip movements
   ■ Supporting knee and ankle, move entire leg away from body (abduction), and then
      — Move entire leg toward the body (adduction).
   ■ Turn to face bed. Supporting knee in bent position (flexion), raise knee toward pelvis (hip flexion).

       — Straighten the knee (extension) as you
         lower leg to bed (hip extension).
     ■ With leg extended, roll leg back and forth
      with one hand above resident's knee and
      other on foot. (Rolling leg inward is internal rotation, rolling leg outward is external
      rotation.)

12. Knee
     ■ Flexion and extension are the only knee
      movements. These were done with flexion
      and extension of hip.

13. Ankle
     ■ Bend resident's knee slightly and support
      lower leg with one hand. With other hand,
      bend resident's foot downward (plantar
      flexion) and then
      — Bend resident's foot forward toward
        resident's body (dorsi flexion).
     ■ With resident's leg extended on bed, place
      both hands on resident's foot and move
      foot inward (inversion), and then
      — Move resident's foot outward (eversion).

14. Toes
     ■ Bend (flexion) and straighten (extension)
      each toe.
     ■ Do abduction and adduction with each toe
      as you did with the fingers.

15. Cover resident's leg and move to other side of
    body. Repeat the movements for each joint.

16. Report to nurse if resident complains of pain
    in any joint during the exercises. Report any
    changes in degree of range that resident is able
    to attain.

17. Perform procedure completion actions.

41. RECTAL TUBE AND FLATUS BAG, INSERTING

Purpose of procedure: To reduce amount of flatus (gas) in bowel.

 1. Perform beginning procedure actions.
2. Assemble equipment:
   - ■ Disposable rectal tube and flatus bag
   - ■ Lubricant
   - ■ Tissues
   - ■ Tape
   - ■ Paper towel
   - ■ Disposable gloves
3. Lower head of bed to horizontal position.
4. Assist resident to assume left Sims' position.
5. Put on gloves.
6. Expose only resident's buttocks.
7. Lubricate tip of rectal tube.
8. Separate buttocks, expose anus, ask resident to take deep breath.
9. Insert lubricated tip of rectal tube 2–4 inches.
10. Secure rectal tube in place with small piece of tape (Figure I-22).
11. Remove and discard gloves. Wash hands.
12. Adjust bedding, make resident comfortable. Leave signal cord close at hand.
13. Return to unit in 20 minutes. Wash your hands.
14. Identify resident, screen unit, explain what you are going to do.
15. Put on gloves.

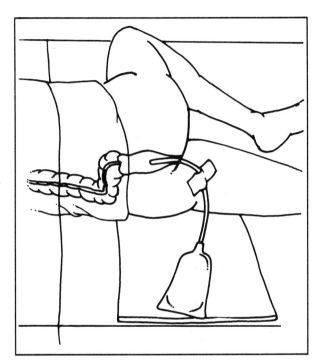

FIGURE I-22. Flatus tube is taped in place for 20 minutes. *(From Caldwell and Hegner,* Nursing Assistant, A Nursing Process Approach, *5th Edition, 1989, Delmar Publishers Inc.)*

16. Gently remove rectal tube, place on paper towel.
17. Remove gloves.
18. Dispose of wrapped rectal tube, bag, and gloves according to facility policy.
19. Perform procedure completion actions.

42. SITTING RESIDENT UP IN BED

Purpose of procedure: To raise resident to sitting position in bed or to raise resident's head and shoulders so pillow can be rearranged.

1. Perform beginning procedure actions.
2. Lock wheels of bed. Place at comfortable working height.
3. Face head of bed. Keep your leg that is farthest away from bed forward. Turn your head away from resident's face. Lock near arms with resident.
4. Support resident with your other arm by making a cradle for resident's head and shoulders.
5. Bring resident to sitting position. Adjust bed position. Rearrange pillows for comfort and support.
6. Perform procedure completion actions.

43. SITTING RESIDENT ON EDGE OF BED

Purpose of procedure: To assist resident to sit on edge of bed before transferring out of bed.

1. Perform beginning procedure actions.
2. Assist resident to turn on side facing you. Have resident flex knees.

3. Place one of your arms under resident's shoulders and the other arm over and around resident's knees.
4. Instruct resident to press down with bottom arm and to use upper arm and hand to press down in order to raise upper body.
5. While resident does this, raise up with your arm that is under resident's shoulders and use your other arm to bring knees off edge of bed.
6. Resident will automatically rise and assume sitting position on edge of bed.
7. Proceed with transfer or ambulation.

 8. Perform procedure completion actions.

44. SITZ BATH, ASSISTING WITH

Purpose of procedure: To apply moist heat to genital and anal area.

 1. Perform beginning procedure actions.
2. Assemble equipment in bathroom:
   - Bath thermometer
   - Bath blanket
   - Disposable gloves if needed
   - Bath towel
   - Clean gown or resident's clothing
   - Safety pin
3. Prepare bath:
   - Check temperature of bathroom. Adjust to 78–80°F.
   - Clean and rinse tub.
   - Fill tub half full. Level of water should extend only to resident's abdomen.

- ▪ Check temperature of water with bath thermometer. It should be 105–110°F.
4. Help resident undress.
5. Put on gloves if resident has perineal pad in place. Remove pad and assist resident into tub.
    - ▪ Some facilities have special tubs for this procedure.
    - ▪ If this is used, resident's feet remain on floor and slippers or shoes can remain on.
    - ▪ Portable units are also available that fit on toilet seat.
6. Cover resident's shoulders with bath blanket. Secure with safety pin.
7. Stay with resident and observe throughout procedure. Discontinue if resident shows signs of fatigue or faintness.
8. Allow some water to run out of tub. Replace it so temperature remains constant. Do not allow hot water to flow directly on resident.
9. Assist resident from tub after 10–20 minutes.
10. Help resident towel dry and put on clean perineal pad if necessary. Remove and discard gloves.
11. Help resident put on clean gown or clothing.
12. Assist resident to return to unit.
13. Clean and disinfect tub.
14. Perform procedure completion actions.

45. SPECIMEN, SPUTUM (Collecting)

Purpose of procedure: To obtain sputum from resident's lungs for testing in the laboratory.

1. Perform beginning procedure actions.

2. Assemble equipment:
    - Container and cover for specimen
    - Requisition and label completed according to facility policy
    - Disposable gloves
    - Tissues
    - Emesis basin
    - Glass of water
3. Put on gloves.
4. Have resident rinse mouth. Use emesis basin for waste.
5. Ask resident to cough deeply to bring up sputum and to expectorate (spit) into container.
    - Have resident cover mouth with tissue to prevent spread of infection.
    - Collect one to two tablespoons of sputum unless otherwise ordered.
    - Do not contaminate outside of container.

(**NOTE:** If 24-hour specimen is being collected, container is left at bedside.)

6. Remove and discard gloves. Wash hands.
7. Cover container tightly and attach completed label and requisition. Place in moisture-proof bag.
8. Promptly take or send specimen to laboratory.
9. Perform procedure completion actions.

46. SPECIMEN, STOOL (Collecting)

Purpose of procedure: To obtain stool for examination for microorganisms, parasites, blood or chemical analysis.

1. Perform beginning procedure actions.
2. Assemble equipment:
   - Bedpan and cover
   - Specimen container and cover
   - Label and requisition completed according to facility policy
   - Toilet tissue
   - Tongue blades
   - Disposable gloves
3. Put on disposable gloves.
4. Give resident bedpan or assist to commode. Instruct resident to avoid urinating if possible when passing the stool.
5. Offer wash water to resident. Take covered bedpan or commode receptacle to utility room or bathroom.
6. Use tongue blades to remove specimen from bedpan or commode receptacle and place in specimen container. Do not contaminate outside of container.
7. Wrap tongue blades in paper towels and discard.
8. Remove and discard gloves. Wash hands.
9. Cover container tightly. Attach label and requisition.
10. Immediately take or send specimen to laboratory.
 11. Perform procedure completion actions.

47. SPECIMEN, STOOL (For Occult Blood Using Hemoccult® and Developer)

Purpose of procedure: To test stool for the presence of blood.

1. Perform beginning procedure actions.
2. Assemble equipment:
    ■ Bedpan with fresh stool specimen
    ■ Hemoccult® slide packet
    ■ Hemoccult® developer
    ■ Tongue blade
    ■ Paper towel
    ■ Disposable gloves
3. Place paper towel on flat surface and open flap of Hemoccult® packet, exposing guaiac paper.
4. Put on gloves.
5. Use tongue blade to take small sample of stool and smear on paper area marked A.
6. Repeat procedure, taking stool sample from different part of specimen and making smear in area marked B.
7. Close tab and turn packet over.
8. Open back tab.
9. Apply two drops Hemoccult® developer directly over each smear. Time reaction.
10. Read results 30–60 seconds later.
11. Presence of blood is indicated by blue discoloration around perimeters of smear.
12. Dispose of specimen.
13. Clean bedpan, dispose of paper towel, packet, and tongue blade.
14. Remove and discard gloves. Wash hands.
 15. Perform procedure completion actions.

48. SPECIMEN, URINE (From Catheter with Drainage Port)

Purpose of procedure: To obtain urine from catheter for examination, without opening drainage system.

1. Perform beginning procedure actions.
2. Assemble equipment:
   - Catheter clamp
   - Completed requisition and label completed according to facility policy
   - Emesis basin
   - 21-gauge or 22-gauge needle
   - Alcohol pads
   - Disposable gloves
   - 10-ml syringe
   - Sterile specimen container and cover
3. Go to bedside 30 minutes before sample is to be collected.
4. Clamp drainage tube.
5. Wash your hands. Return to bedside after 30 minutes.
6. Put on gloves.
7. Place emesis basin on bed under catheter drainage port.
8. Wipe drainage port with alcohol pad.
9. Carefully remove cap on syringe. Do not contaminate tip.
10. Attach needle carefully. Do not contaminate needle.
11. Open package containing specimen container. Remove cover and lay it topside up on bedside stand.
12. Insert needle into port and withdraw specimen (Figure I-23).
13. Carefully withdraw needle.
14. Wipe port with alcohol pad.
15. Transfer urine sample to specimen container.

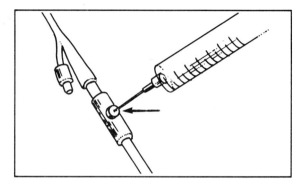

FIGURE I-23. When indwelling catheter has a sample port, syringe is inserted in port to gather specimen. *(From Caldwell and Hegner, Nursing Assistant, A Nursing Process Approach, 5th Edition, 1989, Delmar Publishers Inc.)*

16. Handle cover by top only and place it on container.
17. Remove catheter clamp.
18. Remove and discard gloves. Wash hands.
19. Attach label and requisition to container. Place container in moisture-proof bag. Promptly take or send to laboratory.
20. Dispose of needle and syringe according to facility policy.

(**NOTE:** Needles should not be recapped or clipped. Always report accidental needle stick to appropriate facility authority immediately.)

21. Perform procedure completion actions.

49. SPECIMEN, URINE (From Catheter without Drainage Port)

Purpose of procedure: To obtain urine specimen from catheter by opening drainage system.

1. Perform beginning procedure actions.
2. Assemble equipment:
   - Bed protector
   - Sterile specimen container and cover
   - Label and requisition completed according to facility policy
   - Catheter clamp
   - Disposable gloves
   - Plastic bag
   - Alcohol pads
3. Go to bedside 30 minutes before sample is to be taken.
4. Clamp catheter.
5. Wash your hands. Return to bedside in 30 minutes.
6. Put on gloves.
7. Place bed protector on bed under catheter drainage tubing connection.
8. Place cover of specimen container on bedside stand with inside of cover facing up.
9. Place container upright on bed protector.
10. Wipe area where catheter joins drainage tubing with alcohol pad.
11. Disconnect catheter and tubing. Do not allow either the end of catheter or end of tubing to touch anything.
12. Position catheter tip over specimen container but do not allow it to touch container.

13. With other hand release catheter clamp, allowing urine to flow into container.
14. Place specimen on bedside table, being careful to touch only outside of container.
15. Wipe both ends of connection sites with alcohol pad and reconnect catheter and tubing.
16. Remove and discard gloves. Wash hands.
17. Place cover on container. Attach label and requisition.
18. Promptly take or send to laboratory.

 19. Perform procedure completion actions.

50. SPECIMEN, URINE (Clean Catch)

Purpose of procedure: To obtain urine that is free of contamination for laboratory examination. This test is a culture and sensitivity test done to determine the presence of bacteria in the urine. This is a diagnostic test for urinary tract infections.

 1. Perform beginning procedure actions.
2. Assemble equipment:
    ■ Sterile specimen container with cover
    ■ Disposable gloves
    ■ Label and requisition completed according to facility policy
    ■ Gauze squares or cotton
    ■ Antiseptic solution
    ■ Bedpan or urinal with cover
    ■ Toilet tissue
3. Have container ready. Place cover on bedside table with inside of cover facing up.
4. Put on disposable gloves.

5. Place female resident on bedpan or give male resident urinal.
6. Wash resident's genital area or instruct resident to do so.
   ■ Female residents:
     — Use gauze or cotton and antiseptic solution to cleanse outer folds of vulva (labia) with front-to-back motion.
     — Discard gauze/cotton. Cleanse inner folds of vulva with another piece of gauze and antiseptic solution, again with front-to-back motion.
     — Cleanse middle, innermost area (meatus or urinary opening) in same manner. Discard gauze/ cotton.
     — Keep labia separated so folds do not fall back and cover meatus.
   ■ Male residents:
     — Use gauze/cotton and antiseptic solution to cleanse tip of penis from urinary meatus down, using circular motion.
     — Discard gauze/cotton.
7. Instruct resident to void, allowing first part of urine to flow into bedpan or urinal.
8. Then catch urine stream that follows in sterile specimen container.
9. Allow last portion of urine to escape.
10. Replace sterile cover on urine container.
11. Remove bedpan or urinal and cover. Assist resident to wipe genitalia with toilet tissue.
12. Assist resident to wash hands.
13. With cover tight on specimen container, wash outside of container. Place container in moisture-proof bag.

14. Empty bedpan or urinal. If resident is on I&O, measure contents and add to I&O sheet. Add amount in specimen container.
15. Remove and discard gloves. Wash hands.
16. Promptly take or send specimen to laboratory with label and requisition attached.
 17. Perform procedure completion actions.

51. SPECIMEN, URINE (Fresh Fractional)

Purpose of procedure: To collect urine specimen for testing for sugar and ketones (acetone).

 1. Perform beginning procedure actions.
2. Assemble equipment:
   - Two specimen containers
   - Urinal or bedpan
   - Testing materials if needed
   - Small plastic bag or paper towels for used toilet tissue
   - Toilet tissue
   - Disposable gloves
3. Go to resident about one hour before test is due. Instruct resident that two samples will be taken: one now and a smaller one in one hour or less.
4. Place resident on bedpan or give urinal.
5. Put on disposable gloves.
6. Encourage resident to urinate. Assist to wipe genitalia. Discard toilet tissue in plastic bag or paper towels and discard.
7. Take bedpan or urinal to bathroom or utility room.

8. Pour sample in one specimen container. Test this sample in case resident fails to void second specimen.
9. Make note of test results but do not record.
10. Measure urine if resident is on I&O and discard.
11. Clean equipment and return to proper area.
12. Remove and discard gloves. Wash your hands.
13. Encourage resident to drink water, if permitted. Record intake if resident is on I&O. Tell resident when you will return for second sample.
14. Return to bedside. Perform beginning procedure actions.
15. Repeat steps 4–12. Record results of test.
16. Perform procedure completion actions.

52. SPECIMEN, URINE (24-Hour)

Purpose of procedure: To collect urine over a 24-hour period for laboratory examination.

1. Perform beginning procedure actions.
2. Assemble equipment:
   - 24-hour specimen container and cover
   - Label and requisition completed according to facility policy
   - Sign for resident's bed
   - Disposable gloves
   - Bedpan or urinal
   - Toilet tissue

3. Emphasize to resident the need for saving all urine that is passed. Place specimen collection container in bathroom in pan of ice.
4. Put on gloves.
5. Place resident on bedpan, give urinal, or assist to commode.
   - ■ Measure and record amount if resident is on I&O.
   - ■ Discard urine.
   - ■ Note date and time of voiding. This time marks the start of the 24-hour collection.
6. Place sign on resident's bed to alert other staff that 24-hour specimen is being collected.
7. All urine that is voided for 24 hours is poured in specimen container. Check facility policy for handling of specimen container (Figure I-24).
8. At end of 24-hour period, ask resident to void one last time. Add this urine to specimen container.
9. Remove and discard gloves. Wash hands.
10. Remove sign from resident's bed.
11. Promptly take or send specimen to laboratory with label and requisition attached.

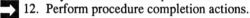

12. Perform procedure completion actions.

53. SUPPOSITORY, RECTAL (Inserting)

Purpose of procedure: To stimulate bowel evacuation or to instill medications. Medicinal suppositories must be inserted by the nurse.

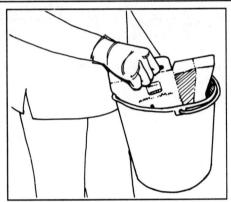

A. The 24-hour urine specimen may require chilling in a bucket of ice.

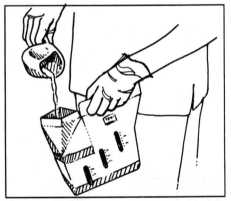

B. Open mouth of container to prevent spilling. Wear gloves to empty urine into container.

FIGURE I-24. The 24-hour urine collection *(From Caldwell and Hegner,* Nursing Assistant, A Nursing Process Approach, *5th Edition, 1989, Delmar Publishers Inc.)*

1. Perform beginning procedure actions.
2. Assemble equipment:
     - Suppository as ordered
     - Toilet tissue
     - Bedpan and cover or bedside commode, as needed
     - Lubricant
     - Disposable gloves
3. Help resident assume left Sims' position.
4. Expose buttocks only.
5. Unwrap suppository and put on gloves.
6. With one hand separate buttocks, exposing anus.
7. Apply small amount of lubricant to anus and insert suppository. It must be inserted deeply enough to enter rectum beyond sphincter muscle (approximately two inches).
8. Encourage resident to take deep breaths and relax until need to defecate is experienced, about 5–15 minutes.
9. Remove and dispose of gloves.
10. Adjust bedding and help resident to comfortable position.
11. Place signal cord within reach and check on resident every five minutes.
12. Position resident on bedpan, commode, or help to bathroom.
13. When resident is finished, put on gloves and assist resident as needed.
14. Assist resident to wash hands.
15. Remove and discard gloves.
16. Report and record results.
17. Perform procedure completion actions.

━━━━━━ **T** ━━━━━━

54. TEMPERATURE, AURAL

Purpose of procedure: To measure body temperature with the infrared tympanic thermometer.

➡ 1. Perform beginning procedure actions.
   2. Assemble equipment:
      - Aural thermometer
      - Probe covers
   3. Place probe cover on probe.
   4. Position plastic probe tip in external auditory canal.
   5. Press button.
   6. Temperature should record in less than two seconds.
   7. Probe cover automatically ejects after each reading.
   8. Record temperature.
➡ 9. Perform procedure completion actions.

55. TOILETING RESIDENTS

Purpose of procedure: To provide residents with a natural method of bowel and bladder elimination.

(**NOTE:** Residents should be taken to the bathroom and toileted, if possible. A commode can be used in resident's room if necessary.)

➡ 1. Perform beginning procedure actions.
   2. Check to see if resident is on:
      - Restorative program for toileting.

- ■Bowel and/or bladder training program.
3. Assemble equipment:
   - ■Wheelchair for nonambulatory resident
   - ■Transfer belt if needed
   - ■Cane or walker if needed for ambulatory resident
   - ■Disposable gloves
   - ■Toilet tissue
   - ■Disposable wipes if needed
   - ■Specimen hat for toilet if resident is on I&O or if specimen is needed
4. If resident is in bed, assist her/him to put on robe. If resident is going to walk to bathroom, be sure resident has shoes and socks on.
5. Have cane or walker in place, if needed. Put transfer belt on resident if needed.
6. If resident cannot walk, place transfer belt on resident and transfer resident to wheelchair (see transfer procedures). Leave transfer belt on resident until resident is transferred to the toilet.
7. Take resident to bathroom. Place specimen hat in toilet if needed. Assist ambulatory resident to sit on toilet. Transfer nonambulatory resident to toilet from wheelchair. Remove transfer belt.

(NOTE: Resident may need help in manipulating clothing before sitting on toilet. If resident needs maximum assistance in transferring, you may need another assistant to help you.)

8. If resident needs assistance to manipulate clothing, take down underwear and slacks while resident is standing. Maintain grasp on transfer belt with one hand and use the other hand to arrange clothing.

9. Be sure resident is comfortable. If resident's feet do not touch the floor, provide a footstool.

10. Provide privacy. Place signal cord within resident's reach if it is safe to leave resident. Check on resident every one to two minutes. If it is not safe to leave, wait discreetly close to resident.

11. Give resident toilet tissue when resident is finished. If resident needs assistance, put on gloves, apply transfer belt and bring her/him to standing position to clean genital area.

12. Assist resident to wash hands.

13. Note character and amount of urine and/or stool.

14. Flush stool unless specimen is needed or urine has to be measured. Remove and discard gloves.

15. Transfer resident from toilet to wheelchair or provide resident with cane or walker if needed.

16. Assist back to room. Assist to remove robe and shoes if resident is going back to bed.

17. Return to bathroom. Put on disposable gloves. Collect specimen, if needed, from specimen hat. Measure urine if necessary and record.

➡ 18. Perform procedure completion actions.

56. TRACTION, CARING FOR RESIDENT

Purpose of procedure: To avoid displacement of fractured bone and to observe for complications associated with traction.

1. Perform beginning procedure actions.
2. Do not disturb weights or permit them to swing, drop, or rest on any surface.
3. Keep resident in good alignment. Make sure body is acting properly as countertraction.
4. Check under belts or straps for areas of pressure or irritation.
5. Make sure straps of halters and belts are smooth, straight, and properly secured.
6. If tongs or pins are placed into bones to hold traction in place, check insertion sites for redness, swelling or drainage. Immediately report these signs to the nurse.
7. If traction is to be discontinued at intervals:
   - Slowly raise weights to bed. Avoid abrupt or jerking movements.
   - If two sets of weights are being used, raise them at the same time and rate of speed.
   - Release weights from connection with halter or belt and place them on floor.
   - To apply traction, reverse procedure.

8. Perform procedure completion actions.

57. TRANSFERRING RESIDENT FROM BED TO CHAIR (One Assistant)

Purpose of procedure: To assist resident to get safely out of bed. This procedure requires only one nursing assistant.

(NOTE: There should be a specific transfer proce-
        dure for each resident who is not an inde-
        pendent, self transfer. Check with nurse or
        care plan for instructions.)

➡ 1. Perform beginning procedure actions.
   2. Assemble equipment:
      ■ Transfer belt
      ■ Chair for resident
      ■ Shoes and socks
   3. Place chair so resident moves toward his/her
      strongest side. Set chair parallel with bed.
      Lock wheels.
   4. Assist resident to sit on edge of bed (see
      Procedure 43).
   5. Give resident time to stabilize and then
      apply transfer belt. Assist resident to put on
      shoes and socks.

(NOTE: Do not allow resident to place hands on
        you while you are transferring. If resident
        is disoriented, becomes frightened, or be-
        gins to fall, he/she may accidentally grab
        your neck or shoulders, causing you seri-
        ous injury.)

   6. If resident has a weak or paralyzed arm, do
      not let it hang or dangle during transfer. Put
      it in his/her pocket or have resident cradle it
      with the strong arm.
   7. When resident is ready to transfer:
      ■ Instruct resident to move forward in chair
        or closer to edge of mattress, to spread

knees, lean forward, and place feet slightly back.

■ If one leg is weaker or should not bear weight, have resident place it in front with strong leg slightly back.

■ Remember to spread your feet apart and bend your knees and hips, keeping your back straight.

■ Hold belt with underhand grasp, one hand on each side of resident.

■ If resident has a weaker leg, press your knee against it or block resident's foot with yours to prevent weaker leg from sliding out from under him/her.

■ Tell resident on count of three to use hands (if able) to press into mattress, straighten elbows, straighten knees, and come to standing position.

8. If resident cannot walk, pivot around to front of chair until chair is touching the backs of his/her legs.

9. Instruct resident to place hands on arms of chair (if able to) and gently lower self into chair as you ease resident down.

10. Position resident comfortably. Place signal light within easy reach.

11. Perform procedure completion actions.

(NOTE: To transfer back to bed, reverse procedure. Chair will need to be turned around so resident moves toward strong side. Or if there is space, move chair to other side of bed.)

58. TRANSFERRING RESIDENT FROM BED TO CHAIR (Two Assistants)

Purpose of procedure: To assist resident to get safely out of bed. This procedure is for a resident who is heavier, taller, has impaired balance, or only partial weight bearing ability.

 1. Perform beginning procedure actions.

NOTE: This procedure is performed the same as the previous one except:

2. Both assistants stand in front of and each to one side of resident.
3. Both assistants put both hands in transfer belt. Each assistant puts outer hand to side and back of resident. The inner hand is placed to side and front of resident.
4. With knees one assistant blocks resident's weak leg (or with foot against resident's foot).
5. On count of three, both assistants and resident pivot around to chair.
6. Continue procedure as with one assistant.
7. Perform procedure completion actions.

59. TRANSFER (GAIT) BELT, APPLYING

Purpose of procedure: To move resident safely and to avoid injury to nursing assistant. Using a transfer belt avoids need to grasp resident around rib cage or under shoulders. Either of these methods can cause serious injury to elderly people.

(**NOTE:** The transfer belt may also be called a gait belt or safety belt. The term gait belt is appropriate when the device is used when ambulating the resident.)

1. Perform beginning procedure actions.
2. Assemble equipment:
   ■ Transfer belt
3. Explain procedure. Tell resident the belt is a safety device that will be removed as soon as resident is safely moved.
4. Apply the belt over resident's clothing. If resident is undressed and being transferred from wheelchair to tub or shower chair, place a towel around resident's waist and then apply belt over the towel.
5. If resident is going to transfer from bed to chair, belt may be applied after resident comes to sitting position on edge of bed. If resident has inadequate balance, belt can be applied while the resident is still lying down in bed.
6. Keep belt at resident's waist level. Avoid placing it too high. Make sure belt is right side out and is not twisted.
7. Buckle the belt in front by threading belt through teeth side of buckle first and then through both openings. Buckle must be in front.
8. Check female residents to be sure breasts are not under belt.
9. Belt should be snug so it doesn't slide up but not too tight.

10. Use underhand grasp when holding belt.
11. Do not overuse belt by pulling resident up with too much force.
12. Belt may be contraindicated for residents with abdominal, back or rib injuries, surgery, abdominal pacemakers, advanced heart or lung disease, or abdominal aneurysms.
13. Remove belt after resident is safely moved.
 14. Perform procedure completion actions.

60. TRANSFERRING RESIDENT FROM BED TO STRETCHER

Purpose of procedure: To move resident to another surface without causing injury to resident or staff. In the long-term care facility, this procedure may be used to move residents from bed to portable bathtub. It may also be used to move a resident onto a prone cart. These are sometimes used for residents who need to lie in prone position. The cart can be wheeled out of the room. The procedure may be very frightening to the resident. Assure the resident that procedure is safe.

1. Perform beginning procedure actions.
2. Assemble equipment:
   ■ Stretcher
   ■ Bath blanket
3. Lock wheels of bed. Raise bed to horizontal position equal to height of stretcher. Lower siderails.
4. Place bath blanket over resident and fanfold top covers to foot of bed, out of the way.

5. You will need people for these positions:
   - ■One assistant against opposite side of bed.
   - ■One assistant at foot of bed, facing head of bed.
   - ■Third assistant against stretcher.
   - ■Fourth assistant at head of bed facing foot.
6. Loosen turning sheet on both sides of bed and roll it against resident.
7. Position stretcher close to bed. Lock stretcher wheels.
8. At prespecified signal, all assistants act together:

(**NOTE:**   Assistant on opposite side of bed may need to kneel on bed to avoid overstretching the back.)

   - ■Assistant at foot of bed lifts resident's feet and legs.
   - ■Assistant against side of bed lifts and guides resident's body with turning sheet.
   - ■Assistant against stretcher grasps turning sheet with both hands, raises, and draws resident onto stretcher.
   - ■Assistant at head of bed cradles resident's head and neck with hands under shoulders, arms together.

9. Center resident on stretcher. Secure stretcher safety belt. Raise siderails of stretcher.
10. Transport resident as directed.
11. Perform procedure completion actions.

61. TRANSFERRING RESIDENT FROM STRETCHER TO BED

Purpose of procedure: To move resident safely from one surface to another. This procedure may be frightening to resident so be sure to assure resident that he/she will be safe.

1. Perform beginning procedure actions.
2. No additional equipment is needed.
3. Lock wheels of bed. Raise bed to horizontal position equal to height of stretcher. Lower siderails. Fanfold bedding to foot of bed.
4. You will need assistants for these positions:
   - One assistant against opposite side of bed.
   - One assistant at foot of stretcher, facing head of stretcher.
   - Third assistant against stretcher.
   - Fourth assistant at head of stretcher, facing foot.
5. Lower siderails of stretcher. Place stretcher parallel to and against bed. Lock wheels of stretcher. Be sure everyone is in position. Remove stretcher safety belt.
6. Loosen turning sheet and roll it against resident.
7. At prespecified signal, all assistants act together:
   - Assistant at foot of stretcher lifts resident's feet and legs.
   - Assistant on opposite side of bed uses both hands to grasp turning sheet. It may

be necessary for assistant to kneel on bed
to lift and draw resident onto bed.

■ Assistant at head of stretcher cradles
resident's head and neck with hands under shoulders and arms together.

■ Assistant opposite stretcher grasps turning sheet to guide resident. All assistants
coordinate their activities and move together.

8. Move stretcher out of way.

9. Use turning sheet to position resident in bed.

10. Pull top covers up over resident. Remove
bath blanket.

 11. Perform procedure completion actions.

62. URINARY CONDOM, REPLACING

Purpose of procedure: To provide a method of external catheter drainage for incontinent male residents. Condom is applied to penis. Drainage tubing is connected to other end of condom for collection in drainage container.

1. Perform beginning procedure actions.
2. Assemble equipment:
   - Basin of warm water
   - Washcloth
   - Condom with drainage tip
   - Disposable gloves
   - Bed protector/bath blanket
   - Plastic bag
   - Towel
   - Paper towels
3. Arrange equipment on over-bed table.
4. Lower siderail on side you are working.
5. Cover resident with bath blanket and fanfold bedding to foot of bed. Place bed protector under resident's hips.
6. Adjust bath blanket to expose genitals only.
7. Put on gloves.
8. Remove old condom by rolling toward tip of penis. Place in plastic bag if disposable. If reusable, put on paper towels to be washed and dried.
9. Wash and dry penis. Observe for signs of irritation.

10. Remove paper from "ready-stick" surface.
11. Apply fresh condom and drainage tip to penis by rolling it toward base of penis. If resident is uncircumcized, be sure foreskin remains in good position.
12. Reconnect drainage system.
13. Remove and discard gloves. Wash hands.
14. Perform procedure completion actions.

63. URINE, STRAINING

Purpose of procedure: Urine is strained when resident is suspected of having kidney stones.

1. Perform beginning procedure actions.
2. Assemble equipment:
    - Bedpan, urinal, drainage bag, or commode receptacle with urine
    - Graduated pitcher, gauze, and rubber band or,
    - Filter paper, funnel, and graduated pitcher
    - Disposable gloves
3. Place gauze over top of graduated pitcher and secure with rubber band (Figure I-25) or
4. Place filter paper in funnel and place in graduated pitcher.
5. Pour urine through gauze or filter paper.
6. Inspect carefully for stones. If present, check with nurse for further instructions. If no stones are present, discard urine.
7. Clean urine receptacle according to facility procedure.
8. Remove and discard gloves. Wash hands.
9. Perform procedure completion actions.

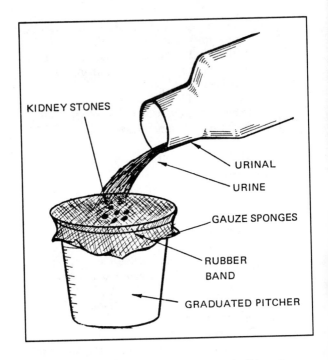

FIGURE I-25. Straining urine through gauze for kidney stones *(From Caldwell and Hegner,* Nursing Assistant, A Nursing Process Approach, *5th Edition, 1989, Delmar Publishers Inc.)*

64. VAGINAL DOUCHE, UNSTERILE

Purpose of procedure: To clean vaginal area; to prevent odors; to prevent infection.

1. Perform beginning procedure actions.
2. Assemble equipment:
   - Disposable douche set
   - Bed protector
   - Toilet tissue
   - Bath blanket
   - Monel cup with cotton balls and disinfectant
   - Irrigating standard
   - Disposable gloves
   - Bedpan and cover
   - Paper bag
3. Pour small amount of specified disinfectant solution over cotton balls in Monel cup.
4. Hang douche bag on standard. Close clamp on tubing. Leave protector on sterile tip.
5. Measure water in douche container. Temperature should be 105°F. Add powder or solution as ordered.
6. Assemble remaining equipment on bedside table.
7. Wash hands again and put on gloves.
8. If perineal pad is in place, remove from front to back and discard in paper bag.

9. Place bedpan under resident and ask her to void. Empty bedpan. Wipe genitalia with toilet tissue. Allow resident to wash and dry hands.

10. Drape resident with bath blanket. Fanfold top bedding to foot of bed.

11. Place bed protector under resident. Place bedpan under resident and assist resident into dorsal recumbent position.

12. Cleanse perineum:
    ■ Use one cotton ball with disinfectant for each stroke.
    ■ Cleanse from vulva toward anus.
    ■ Cleanse labia majora first.
    ■ Expose labia minora with thumb and forefinger and cleanse.
    ■ Give special attention to folds.
    ■ Discard cotton balls in emesis basin.

13. Open clamp to expel air. Remove protector from sterile tip of disposable douche.

14. Allow small amount of solution to flow and insert nozzle slowly and gently into vagina with upward and backward movement for about three inches.

15. Rotate nozzle from side to side as solution flows.

16. When all solution has been given, remove nozzle slowly and clamp tubing.

17. Assist resident to sit up on bedpan to allow all solution to return.

18. Remove douche bag from standard and place on paper towels.

19. Dry perineum with tissue and discard in bedpan.
20. Cover bedpan and place on chair.
21. Have resident turn on side. Dry buttocks with tissue.
22. Place clean perineal pad (if required) over vulva from front to back.
23. Remove bed protector and bath blanket. Replace with top bedding.
24. Observe contents of bedpan. Note character and amount of discharge, if any. Discard contents.
25. Clean bedpan.
26. Remove and discard gloves. Wash hands.
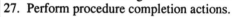 27. Perform procedure completion actions.

65. WARM ARM SOAK

Purpose of procedure: To apply moist heat to arm and hand.

1. Perform beginning procedure actions.
2. Assemble equipment:
   - Bath thermometer
   - Arm-soak basin
   - Pitcher
   - Large plastic sheet
   - Bath towel
   - Bath blanket
3. Bring equipment to bedside.
4. Cover resident with bath blanket. Fanfold bedding to foot of bed.
5. Expose arm to be soaked. Elevate head of bed to sitting position, if allowed.
6. Help resident move to far side of bed. Be sure siderail is up and secure.
7. Cover bed with plastic sheet and towel.
8. Fill arm-soak basin half full with 100°F water. Check with bath thermometer.
9. Place basin on bed protector and assist resident to gradually place arm in basin.
10. Check temperature every five minutes. Use pitcher to get additional water and add to basin to maintain temperature.
11. Discontinue procedure at end of prescribed time.

■ Lift arm out of basin.
■ Slip basin forward and allow arm to rest on bath towel.
■ Place basin on over-bed table. Pat arm dry with towel.

12. Remove plastic sheet and towel.
13. Adjust bedding and remove bath blanket.
14. Lower head of bed and make resident comfortable.
15. Clean and store equipment according to facility policy.

 16. Perform procedure completion actions.

66. WARM FOOT SOAK

Purpose of procedure: To apply moist heat to foot.

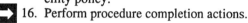 1. Perform beginning procedure actions.
2. Assemble equipment:
    ■ Bath thermometer
    ■ Pitcher
    ■ Solution as ordered, in container
    ■ Large plastic sheet
    ■ Tub or basin of appropriate size
    ■ Two bath blankets
    ■ Two bath towels
3. Have resident flex knees. Loosen top bedding at foot of bed and fold back.
4. Place plastic sheet across foot of bed. Cover with bath blanket, folded in half, with top half fanfolded toward foot of bed.
5. Place towel on blanket and hot water bottle at lower edge of towel.

6. Raise resident's feet. Draw plastic sheet, blanket, and bath towel up under legs and feet. Bring upper half of bath blanket over feet.

7. Fill tub half full of water about 100°F. Place at foot of bed.

8. Raise resident's feet with one hand, draw tub under them and gradually immerse one or both feet as ordered. Place towel between edge of tub and legs.

9. Draw bath blanket up over knees and fold it over from each side. Bring top covers over foot of bed.

10. Replenish water to maintain temperature.

11. Discontinue treatment within 15–20 minutes.

12. Remove feet from tub and move them to towel with hot water bottle under towel. Cover feet.

13. Remove tub to table or chair.

14. Dry feet. Remove hot water bottle.

15. Remove bath blanket, plastic sheet, and towel.

16. Draw down top covers and tuck in at foot.

17. Clean and store equipment according to facility policy.

18. Perform procedure completion actions.

67. WARM WATER BAG

Purpose of procedure: To apply dry heat to a specific body part.

1. Perform beginning procedure actions.
2. Assemble equipment:
   - ■ Hot water bottle
   - ■ Paper towels
   - ■ Bath thermometer
   - ■ Container for hot water, or use sink
   - ■ Cotton cover for hot water bottle
3. Prepare hot water bottle:
   - ■ Fill container with water about 115°F. (Use thermometer.)
   - ■ Fill bottle one-third to one-half full.
   - ■ Expel air; place bottle horizontally on flat surface; hold neck of bottle upright until water reaches top. Close top.
4. Wipe bottle dry with paper towels. Turn upside down to check for leaks.
5. Cover bag with cotton cover.
6. Take to bedside.
7. Place bag to area as ordered. Do not allow resident to lie on bag.
8. Check resident at frequent intervals. Report unusual observations to nurse.
9. Repeat procedure as ordered.
10. Clean and store equipment according to facility procedure.
11. Perform procedure completion actions.

68. WEIGHING AND MEASURING RESIDENT IN BED

Purpose of procedure: To monitor resident's nutritional status and fluid balance by measuring body size. This procedure is used for the resident who is unable to stand on an upright scale.

1. Perform beginning procedure actions.
2. Assemble equipment:
   - Over-bed scale
   - Tape measure
   - Pencil
3. Obtain assistance.
4. Check scale sling and straps for frayed areas or poorly closing straps.
5. Lower siderail on your side. Make sure siderail on other side is up.
6. Position resident flat on back with arms and legs straight.
7. Make small pencil mark at top of resident's head on sheet.
8. Make second pencil mark even with feet.
9. Using tape measure, measure distance between two marks.
10. Note this on pad as resident's height in feet and inches, or in centimeters, according to facility policy.
11. Remove scale sling and position half under resident.
    - Turn resident away from you.
    - Place sling folded lengthwise under resident.
    - Turn resident toward you and position sling so resident rests securely within it.
    - Attach sling to suspension straps. Check to be sure attachments are secure.

12. Position lift frame over bed with base legs in maximum open position and lock.
13. Elevate head of bed and bring resident to sitting position.
14. Attach suspension straps to frame. Position resident's arms inside straps.
15. Raise sling so resident's body is free from bed.
16. Guide lift away from bed so no part of resident touches bed.
17. Adjust weights to balance scale.
18. Take and note reading.
19. Reposition sling over center of bed.
20. Release knob slowly, lowering resident to bed.
21. Remove sling by reversing process in Step 11.
22. Assist resident into comfortable position.
23. Move over-bed scale out of way.
24. Raise siderail and lower bed to lowest horizontal position.
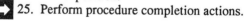
25. Perform procedure completion actions.

Glossary

abduction – movement away from midline of center.

abuse – to mistreat.

activities of daily living (ADL) – activities that help residents fulfill their basic human needs.

adaptive equipment – items used for activities of daily living that have been altered for use by individuals with disabilities.

adduction – movement toward midline or center.

ADL – activities of daily living.

aged – old; usually refers to those over 75 years of age.

aging – natural, progressive process that begins at birth.

alert – mentally responsive.

alignment – proper position.

aneurysm – blood-filled sac formed by dilation of the walls of a blood vessel, usually an artery.

anger – state of grieving when a patient is no longer able to deny awareness of a terminal diagnosis and exhibits feelings of frustration.

anus – outlet of the rectum lying in fold between the nates.

aphasia – language impairment.

artery – vessel through which blood passes away from heart to various parts of body.

articulation – ability to express oneself clearly.

aspiration – drawing of foreign material into respiratory tract.

assault - attempt or threat to do violence to another.

assistive devices – objects used to help an individual ambulate, such as canes, crutches, and walkers.

atrophy – shrinking or wasting away of tissues.

chart – record of information concerning a patient.

colon – another name for the large intestine.

colostomy – artificial opening in abdomen for purpose of evacuation.

communicable – transmissible from person to person, such as from an infectious disease.

communication – passage of a message from a sender to a receiver.

confidential – keeping what is said or written to oneself.

confusion – disturbed orientation concerning time, place, or person; sometimes accompanied by disorientated consciousness.

contaminated – unclean; carrying germs.

contracture – permanent contractions of a muscle due to spasm or paralysis.

cyanosis – bluish skin discoloration due to lack of oxygen.

decubitus – pressure sore.

decubitus ulcer – bedsore or pressure sore.

dementia – progressive mental deterioration due to organic disease of brain.

depression – feelings of sadness; one of the stages of grieving.

disability – physical or mental restriction or disadvantage.

disorientation – loss or recognition of time, place, or person.

displacement – defense mechanism in which an emotion is shifted from its real cause to a more acceptable one.

disposable – not reusable.

dyspnea – difficult or labored breathing.

edema – excessive accumulation of fluid in tissues.

elimination – discharge from body of indigestible material and of waste products of body metabolism; excretion.

expiration – expulsion of air or other vapor from lungs.

extension – two ends of any jointed part moving away from each other; to increase the angle between two bones.

flatus – gas or air in stomach or intestine.

flexion – decreasing the angle between two bones.

flow rate – rate at which a fluid moves.

functional – useful.

genitals – sexual organs.

geriatrics – care of the elderly.

gerontology – study of the aging process.

hygiene – system of rules designed to promote health.

ileostomy – a surgical operation in which part of small intestine (ileum) is brought through abdominal wall to create an artificial opening through which feces is eliminated.

incident – occurrence.

incontinence – inability to resist urge to defecate or urinate.

infectious – capable of causing infection.

intravenous infusion – nourishment given through a sterile tube into the veins; also injection of a solution, such as medication, to secure an immediate result.

isolation – place where residents with easily transmitted diseases are kept separate from other patients.

isolation technique – name given to method of caring for residents with easily transmitted diseases.

living will – will written by a terminally ill resident expressing the wish that no extraordinary means be employed to prolong life.

maladaptive – inappropriate reactions due to mental breakdown.

manipulative – dealing shrewdly with others in order to gain attention.

mitered corner – one type of corner used in making a facility bed.

mobility – ability to move about.

nasogastric tube – tube inserted in nose and extending into stomach.

negligence – failure to give the care that can reasonably be expected.

nutrition – process by which body uses food for growth and repair and to maintain health.

palmer flexion – bending of wrist downward.

paralysis – loss or impairment of ability to move part of the body.

plantar flexion – pointing of toes downward.

projection – attributing one's own unacceptable feeling and thoughts to others.

psychosocial – psychological and social.

reaction formation – repressing reality of a situation and then exhibiting behaviors that are opposite of real feelings.

reality orientation – technique of assisting residents to become more aware of their surroundings or environment.

rectum – lower part of large intestine, about five inches long, between sigmoid flexure and anal canal.

repression – unconsciously refusing to recognize a painful thought, memory, feeling, or impulse.

resident – person who needs health care in a long-term care facility.

resident care plan – written, detailed program of care to be given to a specific resident.

residents' rights – list of standards, treatments, and care to which a resident is entitled.

seizure – sudden attack.

shearing force – damaging pressure that occurs as weight of torso and gravity tend to pull deep tissues such as muscle and bone in one direction while skin tends to remain stationary.

signs and symptoms – objective and subjective indications of disease.

spasticity – resistance to passive movement of a limb.

sphygmomanometer – instrument for determining arterial pressure; blood pressure gauge.

stethoscope – instrument used in auscultation to convey to ear the sounds produced in body.

stoma – artificial, mouthlike opening.

suppository – device used to help bowels eliminate feces.

suppression – deliberately (consciously) refusing to recognize a painful thought, memory, feeling, or impulse.

systolic – blood pressure reading taken when pressure is greatest, during contractions; refers to contraction phase of cardiac cycle.

tremors – a rhythmical movement, usually of head, hands, or feet.

trochanter roll – rolled towel or bath blanket placed against lateral thigh to maintain proper alignment.

vomitus – matter ejected from stomach through mouth.

Index

NOTES